THE PANCREATITIS DIET COOKBOOK

Nourishing Recipes for Managing Inflammation"

Disa Sophie

Table of Contents

INTRODUCTION

Understanding Pancreatitis and the Importance of Diet.

Pancreatitis is a medical illness that develops when the pancreas, a critical organ found beneath the stomach, becomes inflamed. The pancreas is important for manufacturing digestive enzymes and hormones that regulate blood sugar levels.

There are two forms of pancreatitis: acute and chronic. Acute pancreatitis is a sudden and severe inflammation of the pancreas, which can be caused by a range of factors such as gallstones, excessive triglyceride levels, alcohol intake, and certain drugs. The symptoms of acute pancreatitis include severe abdominal pain, nausea, vomiting, and fever. Acute pancreatitis can be treated with hospitalization and can be resolved within a few days with correct treatment.

Chronic pancreatitis, on the other hand, is a long-term illness caused by repeated bouts of acute pancreatitis. It can lead to irreversible damage to the pancreas and result in malabsorption, diabetes, and chronic pain. The symptoms of chronic pancreatitis may be similar to those of acute pancreatitis, but they are usually less severe and may be persistent for a longer period of time.

Risk factors for pancreatitis include heavy alcohol intake, gallstones, high triglyceride levels, and certain medical diseases such as cystic fibrosis and high calcium levels in the blood. It's also crucial to know that certain drugs can raise the risk of pancreatitis, such as azathioprine, 6-mercaptopurine, and methotrexate.

The diagnosis of pancreatitis usually involves a physical examination, laboratory tests, and imaging techniques such as an ultrasound, CT scan, or MRI. It is crucial to diagnose and treat pancreatitis as quickly as possible to prevent irreparable damage to the pancreas.

Treatment of pancreatitis often entails hospitalization and supportive treatment, such as pain control and fluid replacement. In situations of acute pancreatitis, therapy may also involve medications to prevent infection and surgery to remove gallstones or drain fluid that has built up in the pancreas. In cases of chronic pancreatitis, treatment may include long-term management of pain and diabetes, as well as diet and lifestyle adjustments to minimize inflammation and prevent future damage to the pancreas.

Diet has a significant role in the management of pancreatitis. When the pancreas is inflamed, it can be difficult to digest food, and consuming the wrong types of foods can make symptoms worse. In the acute phase of pancreatitis, patients are often placed on a clear liquid diet to give the pancreas a chance to rest and heal. As symptoms improve, patients may be able to gradually introduce more solid meals to their diet, but it is vital to avoid foods that can irritate the pancreas, such as high-fat foods, spicy foods, and alcohol.

For chronic pancreatitis, maintaining a nutritious diet is vital to managing symptoms and preventing complications. A diet low in fat and high in fiber can help reduce inflammation and improve digestion. It is also crucial to monitor blood sugar levels and control any diabetes that may develop as a result of chronic pancreatitis. A licensed dietician can work with patients to establish a personalized food plan that matches their specific needs.

It is also vital for individuals with pancreatitis to maintain a healthy weight, as obesity is a risk factor for developing pancreatitis. Regular exercise and avoiding smoking can also help minimize the chance of problems.

Nutrition plays a crucial role in addressing both acute and chronic pancreatitis. A diet that is low in fat and high in fiber, together with monitoring blood sugar levels, can help manage symptoms and prevent complications. It is crucial to engage with a certified dietitian to design an individualized food plan for the best outcome.

In conclusion, understanding pancreatitis is vital for recognizing the symptoms, risk factors, and right therapy for the condition. Also, the importance of food and lifestyle modifications in controlling the illness can't be stressed enough.

CHAPTER 1

The Pancreatitis Diet: What to Eat and What to Avoid.

A low-fat and high-fiber diet.

The pancreatitis diet is a dietary therapy that tries to control the symptoms of pancreatitis and prevent complications. The diet is supposed to be low in fat and high in fiber, with a focus on nutrient-dense foods that are easy to digest. It is also vital to avoid items that can irritate the pancreas, such as high-fat foods, spicy foods, and alcohol.

A licensed dietician can work with patients to establish a personalized food plan that matches their specific needs. In addition to diet, it is also vital for individuals with pancreatitis to maintain a healthy weight, as obesity is a risk factor for developing pancreatitis.

Nutrient-dense foods that are easy to digest.

Examples of nutrient-dense foods that are easy to digest include lean protein sources, whole grains, fruits, and vegetables. These foods can contain crucial vitamins, minerals, and antioxidants that are important for healing and overall health.

Lean protein sources such as fish, chicken, turkey, and tofu are easy to digest and can provide the body with the required building blocks for healing and repair. For example, a person with pancreatitis can have grilled or baked fish, skinless chicken breast, or tofu stir fry with veggies like broccoli, carrots, and bell peppers.

Whole grains such as quinoa, brown rice, and oats are very easy to digest and include key nutrients such as fiber, B vitamins, and minerals. A person with pancreatitis can have quinoa and vegetable salad, brown rice and vegetable stir fry, or oatmeal with fruits like berries, bananas, and honey.

Fruits and vegetables are particularly vital for a pancreatitis diet as they are high in vitamins, minerals, and antioxidants. These meals can be easily digestible if they are prepared or mixed. For example, a person with pancreatitis can take a smoothie prepared with fruits like berries, bananas, and spinach or carrot and ginger soup.

It's crucial to remember that while some foods may be easier to digest, it's important to monitor the symptoms and alter the diet accordingly. Some patients may find that specific fruits and vegetables cause discomfort, so it's vital to be careful of this and make adjustments as needed. It's always better to contact a qualified dietitian to help design a tailored diet plan that is suited for the unique needs of the patient.

High-fat foods, fried foods, spicy foods, and alcohol.

There are certain foods that should be avoided when following a pancreatitis diet, such as high-fat foods, fried foods, spicy foods, and alcohol. These foods can irritate the pancreas and make symptoms worse.

High-fat foods such as red meats, butter, cheese, and fried foods should be avoided. These foods can be difficult to digest and put extra stress on the pancreas. For example, a person with pancreatitis should avoid foods like burgers, fried chicken, bacon and fatty cuts of meat.

Fried foods should also be avoided as they are high in fat and can be difficult to digest. Fried foods such as French fries, onion rings, and fried chicken should be avoided. Instead, a person with pancreatitis should opt for baked, grilled, or steamed foods.

Spicy foods can also be a problem for those with pancreatitis as they can cause inflammation and irritation of the pancreas. Foods such as hot peppers, hot sauce, and curries should be avoided.

Alcohol consumption should also be avoided as it can cause inflammation and damage to the pancreas. Drinking alcohol can also worsen symptoms of pancreatitis, such as abdominal pain and nausea.

It's important to note that everyone's tolerance for different foods may vary, and it's best to monitor symptoms and adjust the diet accordingly. Some people may find that they can tolerate small amounts of these foods, while others may need to avoid them completely. It's always best to consult with a registered dietitian to help create an individualized diet plan that is appropriate for the specific needs of the patient

The role of a registered dietitian in creating an individualized diet plan.

A licensed dietitian plays a key role in designing a personalized food plan for people with pancreatitis. A registered dietitian is a healthcare professional who is trained in the science of nutrition and can help patients comprehend the relationship between diet and health. They can work with patients to build a food plan that matches their unique needs, taking aspects such as symptoms, medical history, and overall health into account.

For example, a patient with pancreatitis may be placed on a clear liquid diet in the acute phase of the disease to give the pancreas a chance to rest and heal. A trained dietitian can work with this patient to design a plan that includes appropriate clear liquids such as water, broths, and clear juices and can also provide advice on when to transition to a full liquid diet and subsequently to a low-fat, high-fiber diet.

A certified dietician can also work with people who have chronic pancreatitis to help control symptoms and prevent complications. They can help construct a food plan that is low in fat and high in fiber and can also provide information on how to manage blood sugar levels if the patient has developed diabetes as a result of the disease. They can help the patient understand how to make good choices, whether eating out or buying packaged foods, and they can also help the patient maintain a healthy weight through regular exercise and a balanced diet.

They can also provide advice on how to satisfy the patient's specific dietary needs, such as providing guidance on how to fulfill protein requirements or how to manage vitamin deficiencies. They can also help address any other dietary difficulties, such as food allergies or intolerances.

In summary, a registered dietitian plays a key role in designing a personalized food plan for patients with pancreatitis. They can provide recommendations on what to eat and what to avoid and can help patients comprehend the relationship between food and health. They can also provide recommendations on how to meet specific nutritional demands, such as protein requirements or how to manage vitamin deficits. They allow the patient to have a higher quality of life and enhance the overall outcome of the disease.

Maintaining a healthy weight and regular exercise.

Maintaining a healthy weight and getting regular exercise are vital to controlling pancreatitis because they can help reduce inflammation and prevent complications.

Obesity is a risk factor for developing pancreatitis, and being overweight can also make symptoms worse. A healthy weight can help to lessen the stress on the pancreas and prevent inflammation. A certified dietician can work with patients to establish a food plan that aids weight loss in a safe and healthy manner. For example, a patient with pancreatitis can be recommended to focus on nutrient-dense foods that are low in calories and rich in fiber and to make sure they are getting enough protein to preserve muscle mass while losing weight. They can also be encouraged to restrict processed meals and added sugars and to make sure they are getting enough fruits and vegetables in their diet.

Regular exercise is also helpful for controlling pancreatitis since it can help reduce inflammation and improve overall health. Exercise can assist in improving blood sugar control and preventing diabetes, which is a typical consequence of pancreatitis. Exercise can also assist in improving general cardiovascular health, which is helpful for controlling symptoms such as stomach pain and nausea.

For example, a patient with pancreatitis can be encouraged to start with low-impact activities such as walking or swimming. As the patient's condition improves, they can progressively increase the intensity and length of their exercise regimen, under the advice of a healthcare expert. They can also be recommended to practice workouts that target the core and abdominal muscles, as these muscles play a critical role in supporting the pancreas and the surrounding organs.

Maintaining a healthy weight and regular exercise are important in treating pancreatitis. A healthy weight can assist to minimize inflammation and prevent complications, while regular exercise can help improve general health and manage symptoms. A registered dietitian and healthcare provider can work together to establish a plan that encourages weight loss in a safe and healthy manner and to provide direction on safe and suitable exercise routines.

Monitoring blood sugar levels.

Monitoring blood sugar levels is a crucial part of diabetes management, especially if the condition is caused by chronic pancreatitis. One method is to use self-monitoring of blood glucose (SMBG), which includes measuring the quantity of glucose in a drop of blood with a small device called a glucometer.

Here's an example of a real-world circumstance in which SMBG can help a diabetic patient with chronic pancreatitis:

Sara was diagnosed with diabetes as a result of a chronic pancreatitis complication. She was shown how to use a glucometer and told to monitor her blood sugar levels before meals and before going to bed. This enabled her to understand how various foods and activities influenced her glucose levels and modify her insulin dosage accordingly.

Regular visits to a healthcare provider are another crucial component of managing blood sugar levels. They might examine the patient's glucose control and look for any problems. An A1C test, which is a blood test that offers an average of the patient's blood sugar over the last 2-3 months, may also be recommended by a healthcare provider.

It is vital to highlight that managing diabetes caused by chronic pancreatitis involves a team approach as well as a combination of self-management and healthcare practitioner input. To develop an effective treatment plan, the patient should collaborate closely with their healthcare provider.

Avoid smoking.

Tobacco use is a big risk factor for a variety of health problems, including chronic pancreatitis. It is especially risky for people with pancreatitis since it increases the chance of consequences like infection, bleeding, and pancreatic scarring.

Here's an example of a real-life scenario demonstrating the need to stop smoking for people with pancreatitis:

Mary was diagnosed with chronic pancreatitis as a result of her excessive alcohol consumption. Her doctor urged her to stop smoking because it increased her risk of developing difficulties. She followed the advice and quit smoking, which aided her recovery and prevented future damage to her pancreas.

Smoking also raises the risk of developing pancreatic cancer, one of the most aggressive and lethal types of cancer. In fact, smokers are 2-3 times more likely than nonsmokers to acquire pancreatic cancer.

Tom was recommended to quit smoking after being diagnosed with chronic pancreatitis in order to lower his chances of developing pancreatic cancer. He stopped smoking, and his doctor diligently followed him for any signs of cancer, which he happily did not develop.

To effectively control the condition and avoid serious complications, patients with chronic pancreatitis must quit smoking. Nicotine replacement treatment, counseling, and pharmaceuticals can all aid in the cessation of smoking.

Smoking is a substantial risk factor for a variety of health issues, including chronic pancreatitis. Smoking cessation is critical for reducing complications and improving overall health in pancreatitis patients.

Monitor symptoms and adjust the diet accordingly.

It is critical to monitor symptoms and change the diet when dealing with chronic pancreatitis. Chronic pancreatitis can cause symptoms such as abdominal discomfort, diarrhea, and weight loss, which can be triggered by specific meals or dietary categories.

Here's an example of a real-life situation in which monitoring symptoms and modifying the diet are critical for chronic pancreatitis management:

After being diagnosed with chronic pancreatitis, Jack observed that consuming high-fat foods made his symptoms worse, such as abdominal pain and nausea." He collaborated with a dietician to develop a low-fat diet plan that enabled him to better manage his symptoms.

Another critical part of symptom monitoring and diet modification is ensuring appropriate nourishment. Chronic pancreatitis patients may have difficulty digesting certain foods, which can lead to malnutrition. A nutritionist can assist in developing a meal plan that will offer all of the required nutrients for a person with chronic pancreatitis, even if specific foods must be avoided.

Samantha was diagnosed with chronic pancreatitis and discovered that she had difficulty digesting certain foods, resulting in weight loss. She worked with a dietician to develop a specific diet plan that provided her with all of the nutrients she needed, despite the fact that she had to forgo some foods. Her symptoms subsided, and she was able to keep a healthy weight.

It is important to remember that controlling chronic pancreatitis involves a team approach, which includes closely monitoring symptoms and changing the diet as needed, as well as collaborating with healthcare specialists such as a nutritionist and a gastroenterologist to develop a successful treatment plan.

Regular follow up with the healthcare provider.

Regular follow-up with a healthcare provider is a crucial part of controlling chronic pancreatitis. Regular check-ups allow the healthcare professional to monitor the patient's symptoms, look for problems, and make any necessary adjustments to the treatment plan.

Here's an example of a real-life circumstance in which regular follow-up with a healthcare practitioner is critical for chronic pancreatitis management:

David saw his primary care physician every three months after being diagnosed with chronic pancreatitis. His doctor would examine his symptoms, perform any necessary tests, and change his treatment plan as appropriate. This constant monitoring enabled David to better control his health and avoid problems.

The healthcare professional may perform a physical examination, run blood tests, and look for symptoms of inflammation or infection during the follow-up visits. They may also modify the patient's medications, such as pain relievers or enzymes, and give lifestyle advice, such as on food and exercise.

Sophie was diagnosed with chronic pancreatitis and was recommended to see her doctor every three months. Her healthcare professional would verify her blood test results, perform a physical examination, and change her treatment plan as needed during her follow-up visits. She found it quite useful in keeping track of her condition and making necessary adjustments to her medication.

It's important to note that managing chronic pancreatitis requires a team approach, which includes regular check-ins with a healthcare provider, close collaboration with other healthcare providers, such as a dietitian, and making lifestyle changes as needed to effectively manage the condition and avoid complications.

CHAPTER 2

Meal Planning and Preparing for a Pancreatitis Diet

Meal planning and preparation for a pancreatitis diet are critical components of controlling chronic pancreatitis. A pancreatitis diet is often low in fat, high in protein, and simple to digest. This diet can help lessen symptoms and prevent consequences from the illness. Meal planning and preparation entails selecting the appropriate foods, cooking them in an easy-to-digest manner, and organizing meals ahead of time to ensure that the patient receives adequate nourishment.

When planning meals for a pancreatitis diet, it's critical to select low-fat, easily digestible foods. Lean proteins such as chicken, fish, and tofu, as well as fruits, vegetables, and whole grains, fall into this category. High-fat foods, such as fried dishes and red meat, should be avoided since they can aggravate symptoms and cause pancreatic damage.

It is critical to prepare food in a digestible manner. Rather than frying, this could involve steaming, boiling, or baking items. Foods should also be chopped or pureed into little pieces to make them easier to digest.

To make meal planning and preparation easier, plan meals ahead of time and prepare food in bulk. Cooking a large amount of chicken or fish and storing it in the refrigerator, for example, can make it simple to add protein to meals throughout the week. Preparing fruits and vegetables ahead of time and storing them in the refrigerator makes it easier to incorporate them into meals.

It is vital to visit a nutritionist to develop a personalized food plan that addresses the patient's individual needs while taking into account the patient's symptoms, medications, and other medical problems. A pancreatitis diet that is well planned can help minimize symptoms, improve general health, and prevent problems connected with the condition.

Meal planning and preparation.

Meal planning and preparation are critical components of chronic pancreatitis management. A pancreatitis diet is often low in fat, high in protein, and simple to digest. This diet can help lessen symptoms and prevent consequences from the illness. Meal planning and preparation entails selecting the appropriate foods, cooking them in an easy-to-digest manner, and organizing meals ahead of time to ensure that the patient receives adequate nourishment.

When planning meals for a pancreatitis diet, it's critical to select low-fat, easily digestible foods. Lean proteins such as chicken, fish, and tofu, as well as fruits, vegetables, and whole grains, fall into this category. High-fat foods, such as fried dishes and red meat, should be avoided since they can aggravate symptoms and cause pancreatic damage. Eating modest, regular meals throughout the day can also help with symptom management.

When selecting the correct foods, it is critical to prepare them in a digestible manner. Rather than frying, this could involve steaming, boiling, or baking items. Foods should also be chopped or pureed into little pieces to make them easier to digest. Cooking meals at home also allows you to have more control over the ingredients you use and keeps you on track with your diet.

To make meal planning and preparation easier, plan meals ahead of time and prepare food in bulk. Cooking a large amount of chicken or fish and storing it in the refrigerator, for example, can make it simple to add protein to meals throughout the week. Preparing fruits and vegetables ahead of time and storing them in the refrigerator makes it easier to incorporate them into meals.

It is also necessary to consult a dietician in order to develop a customized food plan that suits the patient's individual demands. The dietician can take the patient's symptoms, medications, and other medical problems into account and provide instructions for an easy-to-follow diet that includes all of the patient's required nutrients.

In essence, meal planning and preparation are critical components of chronic pancreatitis management. Patients can lessen symptoms, enhance general health, and avoid complications connected with the illness by following a well-planned diet. It takes a collaborative approach and regular communication with healthcare specialists, such as a nutritionist, to ensure that the patient is receiving sufficient nutrition and making the required dietary adjustments.

Choosing pancreatitis-friendly foods.

The correct foods for a pancreatitis diet are a crucial part of managing the condition. A pancreatitis-friendly diet often consists of lean proteins, fruits, vegetables, and whole grains, with low-fat items avoided.

Lean proteins like chicken, fish, and tofu are ideal for a pancreatitis diet. These proteins are low in fat and simple to digest, which can help alleviate symptoms and avoid consequences. Fish, in particular, is high in omega-3 fatty acids, which have anti-inflammatory qualities and can help lower pancreatic inflammation.

Fruits and vegetables are also essential components of a pancreatitis diet. They are high in vitamins, minerals, and antioxidants, as well as being low in fat and easily digestible. Leafy greens like spinach and kale, as well as citrus fruits like oranges and lemons, are some of the best fruits and vegetables for a pancreatitis diet. Berries high in antioxidants, such as strawberries and blueberries, are also excellent alternatives.

Brown rice, quinoa, and whole wheat bread are other excellent choices for a pancreatitis diet. Whole grains are high in fiber, which can aid in the promotion of regular bowel motions and the prevention of constipation, a typical consequence of pancreatitis. They are low in fat and simple to digest.

High-fat foods, on the other hand, should be avoided on a pancreatitis diet, such as fried dishes, red meat, butter, and full-fat dairy items. These meals are difficult to digest and can aggravate symptoms as well as harm the pancreas. High-fat diets can also raise the risk of problems, including infection and bleeding.

Preparing foods in digestible ways.

Food preparation that is easier to digest is an important element of controlling chronic pancreatitis. Cooking procedures like steaming, boiling, or baking can help make foods more digestible and alleviate symptoms like gut pain and diarrhea.

Steaming is a cooking technique in which food is placed in a steamer basket above boiling water. Boiling water's heat and vapor cook the meal while conserving its nutrients and keeping it moist. Steaming is an excellent method for cooking vegetables, seafood, and poultry since it preserves their natural flavors and makes them easy to digest.

Another method of cooking in which food is placed in a kettle of boiling water is steaming. The heat and water cook the food, and it can be an effective way for cooking grains like rice and quinoa as well as vegetables like potatoes. Boiling also aids in the removal of poisons found on the surface of various fruits and vegetables.

Baking is a dry-heat cooking method in which food is placed in an oven and cooked by the hot air that surrounds it. Baking is an excellent way for preparing lean proteins such as chicken and fish, as well as vegetables such as sweet potatoes. Baking is also a fantastic way to cook grains like brown rice, quinoa, and whole wheat bread.

Frying, sautéing, and roasting, on the other hand, should be avoided since they require high heat and high-fat oils, which can make foods more difficult to digest and increase symptoms. Grilling and barbecuing are also not suggested since they can result in charring and the creation of hazardous chemicals.

Meal planning and preparation in bulk.

Meal planning and preparation in bulk can help with chronic pancreatitis management. Planning meals ahead of time and cooking food in bulk can save time and effort while also ensuring that the patient receives adequate nutrients.

Cooking a large amount of lean proteins, such as chicken or fish, and storing it in the refrigerator is one method of bulk meal planning and preparation. This can make it simple to incorporate protein into meals throughout the week. Cooked chicken or fish can be used in salads, sandwiches, soups, and stir-fries, for example.

Another method for bulk meal planning and preparation is to prepare fruits and vegetables in advance and keep them in the refrigerator. This makes it simple to incorporate them into meals such as salads and stir-fries. You can also purée or slice them and freeze them for later use.

Planning meals ahead of time can also help you ensure that you have all of the necessary components on hand and avoid last-minute treks to the grocery store. Meal planning and preparation in bulk also allows you to regulate portion sizes and have a variety of meals throughout the week.

It's also worth noting that while cooking food in quantity, it's critical to properly preserve the food to avoid spoiling and food-borne infections. It is critical to use airtight containers and keep them in the refrigerator or freezer, depending on the type of food and the length of time it will be stored.

To summarize, meal planning and preparation in bulk can help with chronic pancreatitis management. Planning meals in advance, cooking food in bulk, and properly storing it can save time and work while also ensuring that the patient receives adequate nutrients.

Consulting a dietitian to design a customized diet.

Consulting a nutritionist to develop a specific diet plan is a crucial part of controlling chronic pancreatitis. Based on the patient's unique demands and medical condition, a dietician can advise on what meals to eat and what foods to avoid. They can also assist in ensuring that the patient is receiving adequate nourishment and making any required dietary changes.

When visiting a nutritionist, the patient's medical history, symptoms, medications, and other health issues will be evaluated. The dietician will then design a customized food plan for the patient based on their individual needs. This may include suggestions for a low-fat, high-protein, easy-to-digest diet as well as portion sizes, meal frequency, and cooking methods.

The dietician will also work with the patient to identify any food triggers that may be exacerbating their symptoms and make any required dietary changes. They may also provide instruction and tools on how to read food labels, plan meals, and make smart food choices when dining out.

Furthermore, the dietician will verify that the patient is obtaining all of the necessary nutrients from their diet, even if they must avoid particular items. They can also offer supplements if necessary to ensure that the patient is getting all of the vital nutrients.

A well-planned pancreatitis diet can provide numerous benefits in the management of chronic pancreatitis. Patients can lessen symptoms, enhance general health, and avoid complications linked with the illness by eating a diet low in fat, high in protein, and easy to digest.

One of the primary benefits of a well-planned pancreatitis diet is symptom relief. Symptoms such as abdominal pain and diarrhea might be caused by pancreatic inflammation, which can be increased by high-fat diets. Patients can lessen inflammation in the pancreas and symptoms by eating a low-fat diet. Additionally, an easy-to-digest food might help minimize symptoms like bloating and gas.

Another advantage of a well-planned pancreatitis diet is improved general health. A low-fat, high-protein, fruit-and-vegetable diet can help the body acquire the nutrients it needs to function effectively. This can also boost energy levels and improve general wellness.

A well-planned pancreatitis diet might also help to avoid problems connected with the condition. Inflammation in the pancreas can result in complications such as infection and bleeding.

Patients can avoid these consequences by following a low-fat diet and lowering inflammation. Furthermore, a dietitian can ensure that the patient is getting all of the necessary nutrients from their diet, even if they must avoid specific foods, and can offer supplements if necessary.

In conclusion, a well-planned pancreatitis diet can provide numerous benefits in the management of chronic pancreatitis. Patients can lessen symptoms, enhance general health, and avoid complications linked with the illness by eating a diet low in fat, high in protein, and easy to digest. It is critical to engage with a healthcare professional and a nutritionist to develop a personalized food plan that suits the patient's individual needs, taking into account the patient's symptoms, medications, and other medical problems.

Finally, meal planning and preparation are critical components of chronic pancreatitis management. Patients can lessen symptoms, enhance general health, and avoid complications connected with the illness by following a well-planned diet. It takes a collaborative approach and regular communication with healthcare specialists, such as a nutritionist, to ensure that the patient is receiving sufficient nutrition and making the required dietary adjustments.

A pancreatitis-friendly diet often consists of lean proteins, fruits, vegetables, and whole grains, with low-fat items avoided. Preparing foods in an easy-to-digest manner, such as by steaming, boiling, or baking, can aid in digestion and lessen symptoms. Meal planning and preparation in bulk can save time and effort while also ensuring that the patient receives adequate nutrients.

Working with a dietician to develop a specific meal plan is a crucial part of controlling chronic pancreatitis. The dietician can take the patient's symptoms, medications, and other medical problems into account and provide instructions for an easy-to-follow diet that includes all of the patient's required nutrients.

Meal planning and preparation is an important part of managing chronic pancreatitis, and it necessitates a team approach as well as regular consultation with healthcare providers, such as a dietitian, to ensure that the patient is getting the proper nutrition and making necessary dietary adjustments. Patients can lessen symptoms, enhance general health, and avoid complications connected with the illness by following a well-planned diet.

CHAPTER 3

Breakfast Recipes for Pancreatitis Management.

Breakfast is a vital meal of the day, and it is critical to ensure that the foods ingested at breakfast are acceptable for a pancreatitis diet. A well-planned breakfast may give the body the nutrients and energy it needs to start the day, while also being easy to digest and low in fat.

When dealing with pancreatitis, it's critical to focus on lean proteins, nutritious grains, and fruits and vegetables. These foods are low in fat and easy to digest, and they can offer the body the nutrients it requires to function correctly.

Breakfast recipes for a pancreatitis diet.

It is important to note that each person is unique and their condition may vary, so it is critical to consult with a healthcare provider and a dietitian to develop a personalized diet plan that meets the specific needs of the patient, taking into account the patient's symptoms, medications, and other medical conditions.

Overall, breakfast is a key meal of the day, and it's critical to ensure that the foods ingested at breakfast are appropriate for a pancreatitis diet, supplying the body with the required nutrients and energy to start the day while also being easy to digest and low in fat.

Day 1: Whole Wheat English Muffin

Ingredients:

2 whole-wheat English muffins
1 avocado
2 poached eggs
4 slices of smoked salmon

Instructions:

Preheat your oven to 350°F (180°C) and place the English muffins on a baking sheet. Toast the English muffins in the oven for about 5–7 minutes, or until they are golden brown and crispy. Remove the English muffins from the oven and let them cool for a few minutes. Cut the avocado in half and remove the pit. Scoop out the avocado flesh with a spoon and mash it in a small bowl.

Spread the mashed avocado on top of each English

muffin.

Poach the eggs by adding water to a pot and bringing it to a simmer, then cracking the eggs into the water and cooking them for about 2–3 minutes. Remove the eggs with a slotted spoon and place them on top of the avocado. Add the smoked salmon on top of the eggs. Serve the English muffins and enjoy. Note: You can also add some vegetables like tomatoes and cucumbers to make it more nutritious.

This recipe provides a good source of protein, healthy fats, and omega-3 fatty acids. It's a great option for breakfast, and it's easy to prepare, delicious, and nutritious. Make sure to use the whole wheat English muffins for a healthier option.

Day 2: Veggie Omelette

Ingredients:

2 eggs

1/4 cup diced bell peppers

1/4 cup diced mushrooms

1/4 cup diced onions

Salt and pepper to taste

1 tsp oil or butter

Instructions:

In a small mixing bowl, whisk together the eggs and set aside.

Heat a non-stick skillet over medium heat. Add the oil or butter.

Once the skillet is hot, add the bell peppers, mushrooms, and onions. Cook until they are softened, about 5 minutes.

Season the vegetables with salt and pepper to taste.

Pour the egg mixture over the vegetables. Use a spatula to spread the eggs evenly over the skillet.

Cook the omelette for 2-3 minutes or until the bottom is set and golden brown.

Carefully flip the omelette and cook for an additional 2-3 minutes or until the other side is set and golden brown.

Serve and enjoy!

Note:

This recipe is a suitable for those with pancreatitis management as it is low in fat and high in protein.

You can use any other vegetables that you prefer, but make sure they are low in fat.

You can also use non-stick cooking spray in place of oil or butter to reduce fat content even more.

Day 3: Greek Yogurt with Mixed Berries

Ingredients:

1 cup Greek yogurt

1/2 cup mixed berries (such as blueberries, raspberries, and blackberries)

1 tbsp. honey (optional)

Instructions:

In a small mixing bowl, combine the Greek yogurt, mixed berries, and honey (if using).

Mix well until the berries are evenly distributed throughout the yogurt.

Serve the yogurt and berry mixture in a bowl or glass.

Enjoy your delicious and healthy breakfast!

Note:

This recipe is suitable for those with pancreatitis management as it is low in fat and high in protein.

You can use any other berries that you prefer, but make sure they are low in fat.

You can also skip the honey if you prefer a less sweet taste or if you are watching your sugar intake.

You may use a low-fat Greek yogurt for even less fat content.

Day 4: Smoothie Bowl

Ingredients:

1 banana

1/2 cup frozen berries (such as blueberries, raspberries, and blackberries)

1/2 cup unsweetened almond milk

1/2 cup plain Greek yogurt

1 tbsp. chia seeds (optional)

1 tsp honey (optional)

Instructions:

In a blender, combine the banana, frozen berries, almond milk, Greek yogurt, chia seeds (if using), and honey (if using).

Blend until the mixture is smooth and creamy.

Pour the smoothie mixture into a bowl.

Add your desired toppings, such as fresh berries, nuts, or granola.

Enjoy your delicious and healthy breakfast!

Note:

This recipe is suitable for those with pancreatitis management as it is low in fat and high in protein.

You can use any other fruits that you prefer, but make sure they are low in fat.

You can also skip the honey if you prefer a less sweet taste or if you are watching your sugar intake.

You may use a low-fat Greek yogurt for even less fat content.

You can also use other type of milk such as soy, oat or rice milk.

You can add spinach, kale or any other greens for added nutrition and fiber

Day 5: Whole Wheat Blueberry Pancakes

Ingredients:

1 cup whole wheat flour

1 tsp baking powder

1/4 tsp salt

1 egg

3/4 cup unsweetened almond milk

1 tbsp honey (optional)

1/2 cup fresh blueberries

1 tsp oil or butter (for cooking)

Instructions:

In a large mixing bowl, combine the whole wheat flour, baking powder, and salt.

In a separate mixing bowl, whisk together the egg, almond milk, and honey (if using).

Add the wet ingredients to the dry ingredients and mix until just combined. Gently fold in the blueberries.

Heat a non-stick skillet or griddle over medium heat. Add the oil or butter.

Once the skillet is hot, use a ladle to pour 1/4 cup of batter onto the skillet for each pancake.

Cook the pancakes for 2-3 minutes or until bubbles appear on the surface and the edges start to look set. Flip the pancake and cook for an additional 2-3 minutes or until golden brown.

Repeat until all the batter is used.

Serve and enjoy!

Note:

This recipe is suitable for those with pancreatitis management as it is low in fat and high in protein.

You can use other type of flour such as oat flour or rice flour.

You can also skip the honey if you prefer a less sweet taste or if you are watching your sugar intake.

You can use non-stick cooking spray in place of oil or butter to reduce fat content even more.

You can use any other type of berries that you prefer, but make sure they are low in fat Oatmeal with fruits and nuts

Turkey bacon and egg sandwich

Whole wheat crepes with fruit and yogurt

Day 6: Turkey Sausage and Sweet Potato Hash

Ingredients:

1 tbsp. oil or butter

1/2-pound turkey sausage, diced

1 medium sweet potato, peeled and diced

1/2 cup diced onions

1/2 cup diced bell peppers

Salt and pepper to taste

2 eggs (optional)

Instructions:

Heat a large skillet over medium heat. Add the oil or butter.

Once the skillet is hot, add the turkey sausage and cook until browned, about 5 minutes.

Remove the turkey sausage from the skillet and set it aside.

In the same skillet, add the sweet potatoes, onions, and bell peppers. Cook until the vegetables are softened, about 5 minutes.

Season the vegetables with salt and pepper to taste.

Add the turkey sausage back to the skillet and stir to combine.

If desired, you can make 2 wells in the hash and crack an egg into each well. Cover the skillet and cook until the eggs are set, about 3-4 minutes.

Serve and enjoy.

Note:

This recipe is suitable for those with pancreatitis management as it is low in fat and high in protein.

You can use other types of sausage such as chicken or turkey sausage and you can also use other vegetables that you prefer, but make sure they are low in fat.

You can also use non-stick cooking spray in place of oil or butter to reduce fat content even more.

This dish can be served with or without the egg, as per your preference

Day 7: Quinoa and Berry Breakfast Bowl

Ingredients:

1 cup cooked quinoa

1/2 cup mixed berries (such as blueberries, raspberries, and blackberries)

1/4 cup unsweetened almond milk

1 tbsp honey (optional)

1 tbsp chopped nuts (such as almonds, walnuts, or pecans)

1 tbsp chia seeds (optional)

Instructions:

In a medium mixing bowl, combine the cooked quinoa, mixed berries, almond milk, honey (if using), chopped nuts, and chia seeds (if using).

Mix well until the berries are evenly distributed throughout the quinoa.

Serve the quinoa and berry mixture in a bowl.

Enjoy your delicious and healthy breakfast!

Note:

This recipe is suitable for those with pancreatitis management as it is low in fat and high in protein.

You can use any other berries that you prefer, but make sure they are low in fat.

You can also skip the honey if you prefer a less sweet taste or if you are watching your sugar intake.

You can use other type of milk such as soy, oat or rice milk.

You can add other nuts or seeds such as pumpkin seeds, sunflower seeds and flaxseed.

Quinoa is a great source of protein and a good alternative to traditional grains

Day 8: Whole Wheat Blueberry Muffins

Ingredients:

1 and 1/2 cups whole wheat flour

1 tsp baking powder

1/4 tsp baking soda

1/4 tsp salt

1/4 cup honey

1/4 cup unsweetened applesauce

1 egg

1/2 cup unsweetened almond milk

1 tsp vanilla extract

1 cup fresh blueberries

Instructions:

Preheat the oven to 375°F (190°C). Grease a muffin tin or line with paper cups.

In a large mixing bowl, combine the whole wheat flour, baking powder, baking soda, and salt.

In a separate mixing bowl, whisk together the honey, applesauce, egg, almond milk, and vanilla extract.

Add the wet ingredients to the dry ingredients and mix until just combined. Gently fold in the blueberries.

Use a ladle or spoon to divide the batter evenly among the muffin cups.

Bake for 18-20 minutes or until a toothpick inserted into the center of a muffin comes out clean.

Let the muffins cool in the pan for 5 minutes before transferring them to a wire rack to cool completely.

Serve and enjoy!

Note:

You can use other type of flour such as oat flour or rice flour.

You can also use other type of sweetener such as maple syrup or agave nectar.

You can use other type of milk such as soy, oat or rice milk.

You can use any other type of berries that you prefer, but make sure they are low in fat.

Day 9: Scrambled Egg and Spinach Wrap

Ingredients:

2 eggs

1/4 cup diced bell peppers

1/4 cup diced mushrooms

1/4 cup diced onions

Salt and pepper to taste

1 tablespoon oil or butter

2 large spinach wraps

Instructions:

In a small mixing bowl, whisk together the eggs and set aside.

Heat a nonstick skillet over medium heat. Add the oil or butter.

Once the skillet is hot, add the bell peppers, mushrooms, and onions. Cook until they are softened, about 5 minutes.

Season the vegetables with salt and pepper to taste.

Pour the egg mixture over the vegetables. Use a spatula to scramble the eggs until they are cooked through.

Warm the spinach wraps in the microwave for 15–20 seconds or until they are pliable.

Place the scrambled eggs and vegetables in the center of each wrap.

Fold the bottom of the wrap up over the filling, then fold in the sides and roll up the wrap to enclose the filling.

Serve and enjoy.!

Note:

You can use any other vegetables that you prefer, but make sure they are low in fat.

You can also use non-stick cooking spray in place of oil or butter to reduce the fat content even more.

Spinach wraps are a good source of fiber and are lower in calories than traditional flour wraps, but you may use any type of wrap that you prefer.

This wrap can be eaten cold or warm, depending on your preference.

Day 10: Whole Wheat French Toast

Ingredients:

2 slices of whole wheat bread

1 egg

1/4 cup unsweetened almond milk

1 tablespoon honey

1/4 teaspoon cinnamon

1 teaspoon oil or butter (for cooking)

Maple syrup and powdered sugar (optional, for serving)

Instructions:

In a shallow dish, whisk together the egg, almond milk, honey, and cinnamon.

Dip each slice of bread into the egg mixture, making sure both sides are evenly coated.

Heat a nonstick skillet over medium heat. Add the oil or butter.

Once the skillet is hot, add the bread slices and cook for 2-3 minutes per side or until golden brown.

Serve the French toast warm with maple syrup and powdered sugar (if desired).

Enjoy your delicious and healthy breakfast!

Note:

You can use other types of bread, such as multigrain or sourdough bread.

You can also skip the honey if you prefer a less sweet taste or if you are watching your sugar intake.

You can use other types of milk, such as soy, oat, or rice milk.

You can use non-stick cooking spray in place of oil or butter to reduce the fat content even more.

You can also add some fresh fruits, such as berries, bananas, or kiwis, to add some extra flavor and nutrition.

You can also use other types of sweeteners, such as maple syrup or agave nectar.

Day 11: Egg and Vegetable Frittata

Ingredients:

8 eggs

1/4 cup diced bell peppers

1/4 cup diced mushrooms

1/4 cup diced onions

Salt and pepper to taste

1 tablespoon oil or butter

1/4 cup shredded cheese (optional)

Instructions:

Preheat the oven to 375°F (190°C).

In a small mixing bowl, whisk together the eggs and set aside.

Heat a nonstick skillet over medium heat. Add the oil or butter.

Once the skillet is hot, add the bell peppers, mushrooms, and onions. Cook until they are softened, about 5 minutes.

Season the vegetables with salt and pepper to taste.

Pour the egg mixture over the vegetables. Use a spatula to spread the eggs evenly over the skillet.

If desired, sprinkle shredded cheese over the top of the eggs.

Place the skillet in the oven and bake for 12–15 minutes, or until the eggs are set and the top is golden brown.

Serve and enjoy.

Note:

You can use any other vegetables that you prefer, but make sure they are low in fat.

You can also use non-stick cooking spray in place of oil or butter to reduce the fat content even more.

You can also use low-fat cheese or skip it entirely for even less fat content.

You can also add some herbs, such as parsley, chives, or thyme, to add some extra flavor.

You can slice the frittata and serve it with a salad or whole wheat bread for a complete and well-balanced breakfast.

Day 12: Tofu and Vegetable Scramble

Ingredients:

1/2 cup diced bell peppers

1/2 cup diced mushrooms

1/2 cup diced onions

1/2 cup diced tomatoes

1/2 cup crumbled firm tofu

Salt and pepper to taste

1 tablespoon oil or butter

Instructions:

Heat a nonstick skillet over medium heat. Add the oil or butter.

Once the skillet is hot, add the bell peppers, mushrooms, and onions. Cook until they are softened, about 5 minutes.

Add the diced tomatoes, crumbled tofu, salt, and pepper.

Stir everything together and cook for an additional 5 minutes until the tofu is heated through and the vegetables are cooked.

Serve and eat.

Note:

Tofu is an excellent source of plant-based protein, and it's also low in fat.

You can use any other vegetables that you prefer, but make sure they are low in fat.

You can also use non-stick cooking spray in place of oil or butter to reduce the fat content even more.

You can also add some herbs, such as parsley, chives, or thyme, to add some extra flavor.

You can serve this dish with whole wheat bread or crackers for a complete and well-balanced breakfast.

You can also add some spices, such as turmeric or cumin, to add some extra flavor and color.

Day 13: Yogurt and Berries on Whole Wheat Waffles

Ingredients:

1 cup whole wheat flour

1 teaspoon baking powder

1/4 teaspoon baking soda

1/4 teaspoon salt

1 egg

3/4 cup almond milk, unsweetened

1 tablespoon honey (optional)

1 tablespoon oil or butter (for cooking)

1 cup plain Greek yogurt

1/2 cup mixed berries (such as blueberries, raspberries, and blackberries)

Instructions:

Preheat a waffle maker.

Combine the whole wheat flour, baking powder, baking soda, and salt in a large mixing bowl.

Whisk together the egg, almond milk, and honey in a separate mixing bowl (if using).

Mix the wet and dry ingredients together until barely mixed.

Pour the batter into the waffle iron that has been preheated and cook according to the manufacturer's instructions.

While the waffles are cooking, put the Greek yogurt and mixed berries in a small mixing bowl.

Remove the cooked waffles from the waffle iron and top with the yogurt and berry mixture.

Serve and have fun.

Note:

Other flours, such as oat flour or rice flour, can be substituted.

If you want a less sweet taste or are watching your sugar intake, you can omit the honey.

Other types of milk, such as soy, oat, or rice milk, can be used.

You can also add fresh fruits like berries, bananas, or kiwis to enhance flavor and nutrition.

You can also use a different sort of sweetener.

Day 14: Whole Wheat Banana Bread

Ingredients:

1 pound whole wheat flour

1 teaspoon baking powder

1/4 teaspoon baking soda

1/4 teaspoon salt 1/4 cup honey 1/4 cup unsalted applesauce

1 egg

1/2 cup almond milk, unsweetened

1 tablespoon vanilla extract

1 cup ripe bananas, mashed (about 2-3 bananas)

Instructions:

Preheat the oven to 350 degrees Fahrenheit (180 degrees Celsius). Grease a 9x5-inch loaf pan with cooking spray.

Combine the whole wheat flour, baking powder, baking soda, and salt in a large mixing bowl.

Whisk together the honey, applesauce, egg, almond milk, and vanilla extract in a separate mixing bowl.

Mix the wet and dry ingredients together until barely mixed. Fold in the mashed bananas gently.

Pour the batter into the loaf pan that has been prepared.

Bake the loaf for 40–45 minutes, or until a toothpick inserted into the center comes out clean.

Allow the bread to cool for 5 minutes in the pan before transferring it to a wire rack to cool entirely.

Serve and have fun!

Note:

Other flours, such as oat flour or rice flour, can be substituted.

Other sweeteners, such as maple syrup or agave nectar, can also be used.

Other types of milk, such as soy, oat, or rice milk, can be used.

Other nuts and seeds, such as pumpkin seeds, sunflower seeds, flaxseed, or chia seeds, can be included.

Bananas provide natural sweetness and moisture to the bread, as well as fiber and potassium.

You can also add chocolate chips, almonds, or dried fruits for added taste.

CHAPTER 4

Light and Healthy Appetizers for Pancreatitis

Light and healthy appetizers are an excellent choice for people suffering from pancreatitis. These snacks are often low in fat, high in protein, and simple to make. They are suitable as a snack or as part of a larger meal. Vegetable crudites with a low-fat dip, grilled or baked chicken skewers, shrimp cocktail, and various types of bruschetta or crostini are also popular options.

To make them more appealing, different ingredients, textures, and flavors can be used. They are an excellent way to begin a meal and to keep you full without feeling bloated. They can help lower the risk of pancreatitis symptoms because they are often low in fat.

Ten Light and Healthy Appetizers for Pancreatitis

Grilled Vegetable Skewers:

Ingredients:

1 red bell pepper, cut into 1-inch pieces

1 yellow bell pepper, cut into 1-inch pieces

1 zucchini, cut into 1-inch slices.

1 yellow squash, cut into 1-inch slices

1 red onion, cut into 1-inch pieces

1/4 cup olive oil

1 tablespoon balsamic vinegar

1 teaspoon dried basil

Salt and pepper to taste

Wooden skewers (soaked in water for at least 30 minutes)

Directions:

In a large bowl, mix together the olive oil, balsamic vinegar, dried basil, salt, and pepper.

Add the bell peppers, zucchini, yellow squash, and red onion to the bowl and toss to coat the vegetables in the marinade. Thread the vegetables onto the skewers, alternating between the different types of vegetables. Preheat a grill to medium-high heat. Grill the skewers for 8–10 minutes, turning occasionally, until the vegetables are tender and slightly charred. Serve the skewers as a healthy appetizer or side dish.

Note: This recipe is suitable for individuals with pancreatitis, as it is low-fat and grilled vegetables are an easy-to-digest food.

Cucumber and tomato salad

Ingredients:

2 large cucumbers, peeled and sliced

2 large tomatoes, diced

1/4 cup chopped fresh parsley

1/4 cup chopped fresh mint

2 tablespoons of olive oil

2 tablespoons of lemon juice

1 clove of garlic, minced

Salt and pepper to taste

Directions:

In a large bowl, combine the cucumbers, tomatoes, parsley, and mint.

In a small bowl, whisk together the olive oil, lemon juice, garlic, salt, and pepper to make the dressing.

Pour the dressing over the cucumber and tomato mixture and toss to combine.

Allow the salad to sit for at least 15 minutes before serving to allow the flavors to meld.

Shrimp Cocktail

Ingredients:

1 lb. medium shrimp, peeled and deveined

1/2 cup ketchup

2 tablespoons fresh lemon juice

2 tablespoons chopped fresh parsley

1 tablespoon of horseradish

Salt and pepper to taste

Directions:

Bring a large pot of salted water to a boil. Add the shrimp and cook for 2-3 minutes, until pink and cooked through. Drain and rinse under cold water to cool.

In a small bowl, mix together the ketchup, lemon juice, parsley, horseradish, salt, and pepper to make the cocktail sauce.

Arrange the cooked shrimp on a platter, and serve with the cocktail sauce on the side.

Baked Chicken Skewers

Ingredients:

1 lb. boneless, skinless chicken breasts, cut into 1-inch cubes

1/4 cup olive oil

2 tablespoons of lemon juice

2 cloves of garlic, minced

1 teaspoon dried oregano

Salt and pepper to taste

Wooden skewers (soaked in water for at least 30 minutes)

Directions:

In a large bowl, mix together the olive oil, lemon juice, garlic, oregano, salt, and pepper.

Add the chicken cubes to the bowl and toss to coat the chicken in the marinade.

Thread the chicken onto the skewers.

Preheat the oven to 375°F.

Place the skewers on a baking sheet lined with parchment paper.

Bake for 15-20 minutes, turning occasionally, until the chicken is cooked through and golden brown.

Serve the skewers as a healthy appetizer or side dish.

Antipasto Platter:

Ingredients:

1/2 cup marinated artichoke hearts

1/2 cup marinated mushrooms

1/2 cup marinated roasted red peppers

1/4 cup sliced black olives

1/4 cup sliced green olives

2 oz. prosciutto, thinly sliced

2 oz. salami, thinly sliced

2 oz. pepperoni, thinly sliced

2 oz. provolone cheese, thinly sliced

2 oz. mozzarella cheese, thinly sliced

Fresh basil leaves, for garnish

Directions:

Arrange the artichoke hearts, mushrooms, roasted red peppers, olives, prosciutto, salami, pepperoni, provolone cheese, and mozzarella cheese on a large platter.

Garnish the platter with fresh basil leaves.

Serve the platter as a healthy appetizer or side dish.

Eggplant and tomato caponata

Ingredients:

1 medium eggplant, diced

2 medium tomatoes, diced

1/4 cup diced onion

2 cloves of garlic, minced

2 tablespoons of olive oil

2 tablespoons red wine vinegar

2 tablespoons chopped fresh basil

1 teaspoon sugar

Salt and pepper to taste

Directions:

In a large skillet, heat the olive oil over medium heat. Add the eggplant, onion, and garlic, and cook until the vegetables are tender, about 10 minutes.

Stir in the tomatoes, red wine vinegar, basil, sugar, salt, and pepper.

Simmer the mixture for an additional 10 minutes, until the tomatoes have broken down and the liquid has thickened.

Remove from the heat and set aside to cool.

Serve the caponata at room temperature as a healthy appetizer or side dish.

Chicken or tuna salad

Ingredients:

2 cups shredded cooked chicken breast or drained canned tuna

1/2 cup diced celery

1/4 cup diced red onion

1/4 cup diced red bell pepper

2 tablespoons mayonnaise

2 tablespoons plain Greek yogurt

1 tablespoon Dijon mustard

1 tablespoon fresh lemon juice

Salt and pepper to taste

Lettuce leaves or whole-grain crackers for serving

Directions:

In a large bowl, combine the chicken or tuna, celery, red onion, and red bell pepper.

In a small bowl, whisk together the mayonnaise, Greek yogurt, Dijon mustard, lemon juice, salt, and pepper.

Pour the dressing over the chicken or tuna mixture and toss to combine.

Cover and refrigerate for at least 1 hour to allow the flavors to meld.

Serve the chicken or tuna salad on lettuce leaves or with whole-grain crackers as a healthy appetizer or side dish.

Note:.

 Use low-fat mayonnaise and Greek yogurt; avoid high-fat options. Also, use low-sodium options if possible.

Whipped Feta Dip

Ingredients:

8 oz. feta cheese, crumbled

1/4 cup plain Greek yogurt

2 tablespoons fresh lemon juice

2 cloves of garlic, minced

1/4 cup chopped fresh parsley

Salt and pepper to taste

Pita chips, vegetables, or crackers for serving

Directions:

In a food processor, combine the feta cheese, Greek yogurt, lemon juice, garlic, parsley, salt, and pepper.

Process until the dip is smooth and creamy.

Serve the dip with pita chips, vegetables, or crackers as a healthy appetizer.

Note: This recipe is suitable for individuals with pancreatitis as it is low-fat and high in protein; feta cheese is low in fat compared to other types of cheese, and Greek yogurt is high in protein. Use low-fat Greek yogurt and avoid high-fat options. Also, use low-sodium options if possible.

Grilled halloumi cheese

Ingredients:

8 oz. halloumi cheese, sliced

2 tablespoons of olive oil

1 tablespoon fresh lemon juice

1 teaspoon dried oregano

Salt and pepper to taste

Lemon wedges, for serving

Directions:

In a small bowl, mix together the olive oil, lemon juice, oregano, salt, and pepper.

Brush the halloumi slices with the marinade.

Preheat a grill or grill pan to medium-high heat.

Grill the halloumi slices for 2-3 minutes on each side, until golden brown and slightly crispy.

Serve the grilled halloumi with lemon wedges as a healthy appetizer.

Note: This recipe is suitable for individuals with pancreatitis as it is low-fat and high in protein. Halloumi is a cheese that is high in protein, low in fat and carbs, and easy to digest. It's also gluten-free and vegetarian-friendly. Avoid high-fat options; use low-fat olive oil; and choose low-sodium options if possible.

Ceviche

Ingredients:

1 lb. fresh white fish, diced

1 cup fresh lime juice

1/2 cup fresh orange juice

1/4 cup chopped red onion

1/4 cup chopped cilantro

1 jalapeno pepper, seeded and finely chopped

1/2 teaspoon ground cumin

Salt and pepper to taste

Corn tortilla chips, for serving

Directions:

In a large bowl, combine the fish, lime juice, orange juice, red onion, cilantro, jalapeno pepper, cumin, salt, and pepper.

Cover and refrigerate for at least 2 hours, or until the fish is fully cooked and opaque.

Drain any excess liquid before serving.

Serve the ceviche with corn tortilla chips as a healthy appetizer or side dish.

Chapter 5

Nutritious Soups and Salads for Pancreatitis.

Soups and salads are good options for people with pancreatitis since they contain a good balance of nutrients and are often easy to digest. To avoid flare-ups, use components that are low in fat and easy on the digestive system.

Consider using a clear broth as the base for soups and adding veggies such as carrots, celery, and onions. Lean proteins such as chicken, fish, or tofu can also be used. Avoid using creamy soups or adding high-fat foods such as cream or butter.

Salads can also be a good option, but make sure to use low-fat dressings and avoid high-fat components like cheese and avocado. A basic vinaigrette of olive oil and vinegar can be an excellent option. Greens like lettuce, spinach, and arugula are also low in fat and easy to digest. Adding lean protein, such as grilled chicken or shrimp, can help make the salad more filling.

It is also crucial to note that it is usually preferable to speak with a doctor or a dietitian before making any big changes to your diet, especially if you have pancreatitis. Based on your exact situation, they can prescribe specific foods that are safe for you to consume.

Vegetable and lentil soup

Ingredients:

1 tablespoon oil or butter

1 onion, diced

2 carrots, peeled and diced

2 stalks celery, diced

2 cloves of garlic, minced

1 cup green or brown lentils

2 cups diced tomatoes

4 cups of vegetable broth

1 teaspoon dried thyme

1 teaspoon dried oregano

Salt and pepper to taste

1/4 cup chopped fresh parsley or cilantro (optional, for garnish)

Instructions:

Heat the oil or butter in a large pot over medium heat. Add the onion, carrots, celery, and garlic. Cook until the vegetables are softened, about 5 minutes.

Rinse and drain the lentils, and add them to the pot along with the tomatoes, vegetable broth, thyme, oregano, salt, and pepper.

Bring the soup to a boil, then reduce the heat to low, cover, and simmer for 20–25 minutes, or until the lentils are tender.

Use an immersion blender to puree some of the soup to thicken it, or puree in a blender or food processor.

Adjust the seasonings as needed and bring the soup back to a simmer.

Ladle the soup into bowls and garnish with fresh parsley or cilantro, if desired.

Serve.

Note:

You can use other types of lentils, such as red lentils, yellow lentils, or black lentils.

You can also add any other vegetables that you prefer, but make sure they are low in fat.

You can also use non-stick cooking spray in place of oil or butter to reduce the fat content even more.

You can also use any type of broth that you prefer, such as chicken or beef broth.

You can also add other herbs, such as rosemary or basil, to add some extra flavor.

You can also add some cooked rice, quinoa, or pasta to make it more filling.

This recipe can also be made in advance and reheated for a quick and easy meal.

Chicken and rice soup

Ingredients:

1 tablespoon oil or butter

1 onion, diced

2 carrots, peeled and diced

2 stalks celery, diced

2 cloves of garlic, minced

1 cup long-grain rice

2 cups cooked, shredded chicken

4 cup chicken stock

1 teaspoon dried thyme

1 teaspoon dried oregano

Salt and pepper to taste

1/4 cup chopped fresh parsley or cilantro (optional, for garnish)

Instructions:

Heat the oil or butter in a large pot over medium heat. Add the onion, carrots, celery, and garlic. Cook until the vegetables are softened, about 5 minutes.

Rinse the rice and add it to the pot along with the chicken, broth, thyme, oregano, salt, and pepper.

Bring the soup to a boil, then reduce the heat to low, cover, and simmer for 18–20 minutes, or until the rice is tender.

Adjust the seasoning as needed and bring the soup back to a simmer.

Ladle the soup into bowls and garnish with fresh parsley or cilantro, if desired.

Serve and enjoy!

Note:

You can use any type of broth that you prefer, such as vegetable or beef broth.

Or any other vegetables that you prefer, but make sure they are low in fat.

Use non-stick cooking spray in place of oil or butter to reduce the fat content.

Minestrone Soup

Ingredients:

1 tablespoon oil or butter

1 onion, diced

2 carrots, peeled and diced

2 stalks celery, diced

2 cloves of garlic, minced

1 can diced tomatoes

1 cup green beans, trimmed and cut into 1-inch pieces

1 cup diced zucchini

1 cup diced potatoes

1/2 cup dried small pasta (such as ditalini or elbow macaroni)

4 cups of vegetable broth

1 teaspoon dried thyme

1 teaspoon dried oregano

Salt and pepper to taste

1/4 cup chopped fresh parsley or cilantro (optional, for garnish)

Instructions:

Heat the oil or butter in a large pot over medium heat. Add the onion, carrots, celery, and garlic. Cook until the vegetables are softened, about 5 minutes.

Add the diced tomatoes, green beans, zucchini, potatoes, pasta, broth, thyme, oregano, and salt and pepper to the pot.

Bring the soup to a boil, then reduce the heat to low, cover, and simmer for 20–25 minutes, or until the vegetables and pasta are tender.

Adjust the seasoning as needed and bring the soup back to a simmer.

Ladle the soup into bowls and garnish with fresh parsley or cilantro, if desired.

Serve and enjoy yourself.

Cream of Mushroom Soup

Ingredients:

1 tablespoon oil or butter

1 onion, diced

2 cloves of garlic, minced

1 lb. sliced mushrooms

2 cups vegetable broth

1 cup unsweetened almond milk or low-fat cream

1 teaspoon dried thyme

Salt and pepper to taste

1/4 cup chopped fresh parsley or chives (optional, for garnish)

Instructions:

Heat the oil or butter in a large pot over medium heat. Add the onion and garlic and cook until softened, about 5 minutes.

Add the sliced mushrooms and cook until they release their moisture and are tender, about 8–10 minutes.

Add the vegetable broth, almond milk or cream, thyme, salt, and pepper. Bring the mixture to a simmer.

Use an immersion blender to puree the soup to a smooth consistency, or transfer the soup to a blender and puree in small batches.

Adjust the seasoning as needed and bring the soup back to a simmer.

Ladle the soup into bowls and garnish with fresh parsley or chives, if desired.

Serve and enjoy!

Note:

Use other types of mushrooms, such as shiitake, cremini, or portobello.

Also, you can use other types of milk, such as soy, oat, or rice milk.

If you prefer, add some cooked rice or pasta to make it more filling.

You can also add some herbs, such as parsley, chives, or thyme, to add some extra flavor.

Butternut Squash and Apple Soup

Ingredients:

1 tablespoon oil or butter

1 onion, diced

2 cloves garlic, minced

1 butternut squash, peeled, seeded, and diced

1 Granny Smith apple, peeled and diced

2 cups vegetable broth

1 cup of unsweetened apple juice

1 teaspoon ground cinnamon

1 teaspoon ground nutmeg

Salt and pepper to taste

1/4 cup chopped fresh parsley or cilantro (optional, for garnish)

Instructions:

Heat the oil or butter in a large pot over medium heat. Add the onion and garlic and cook until softened, about 5 minutes.

Add the butternut squash, apple, vegetable broth, apple juice, cinnamon, nutmeg, salt, and pepper. Bring the mixture to a simmer.

Cover the pot and reduce the heat to medium-low; cook until the squash and apples are tender, about 20–25 minutes.

Use an immersion blender to puree the soup to a smooth consistency, or transfer the soup to a blender and puree in small batches.

Adjust the seasoning as needed and bring the soup back to a simmer.

Ladle the soup into bowls and garnish with fresh parsley or cilantro, if desired.

Serve and enjoy!

Note:

You can also use other types of sweeteners, such as maple syrup or agave nectar.

Use other types of milk, such as soy, oat, or rice milk.

Add some cooked rice or quinoa to make it more filling.

Add some herbs, such as parsley, cilantro, or thyme, to add some extra flavor.

You can also add some nuts or seeds, such as pumpkin seeds, sunflower seeds, flaxseed, or chia seeds.

Butternut squash and apple are a great combination of flavors, adding some sweetness and creaminess to the soup and also adding some extra fiber and potassium.

Leek and Potato Soup

Ingredients:

1 tbsp oil or butter

2 leeks, white and light green parts only, cleaned and thinly sliced

2 cloves garlic, minced

2 cups diced potatoes

4 cups chicken or vegetable broth

1 tsp dried thyme

Salt and pepper to taste

1/4 cup chopped fresh parsley or chives (optional, for garnish)

Instructions:

Heat the oil or butter in a large pot over medium heat. Add the leeks and garlic, cook until softened, about 5 minutes.

Add the diced potatoes, broth, thyme, salt and pepper. Bring the mixture to a simmer.

Cover the pot and reduce the heat to medium-low, cook until the potatoes are tender, about 20-25 minutes.

Use an immersion blender to puree the soup to a smooth consistency or transfer the soup to a blender and puree in small batches.

Adjust the seasoning as needed and bring the soup back to a simmer.

Ladle the soup into bowls and garnish with fresh parsley or chives, if desired.

Serve and enjoy!

Note:

Use other type of potatoes such as Yukon Gold or Red Potatoes.

You can also use other type of broth such as chicken or beef broth.

Add some cooked rice or quinoa to make it more filling.

You can also add some herbs such as parsley, chives or thyme to add some extra flavor.

Leek and Potato are a great combination of flavors, adding some sweetness and creaminess to the soup, and also adding some extra fiber and potassium.

Chicken and Vegetable Noodle Soup

Ingredients:

1 tablespoon oil or butter

1 onion, diced

2 carrots, peeled and diced

2 stalks celery, diced

2 cloves garlic, minced

2 cups cooked, shredded chicken

1 cup diced celery

1 cup diced carrots

1 cup diced zucchini

1-pound egg noodles

4 cup chicken stock

1 teaspoon dried thyme

Salt and pepper to taste

1/4 cup chopped fresh parsley or cilantro (optional, for garnish)

Instructions:

Heat the oil or butter in a large pot over medium heat. Add the onion, carrots, celery, and garlic. Cook until the vegetables are softened, about 5 minutes.

Add the shredded chicken, celery, carrots, zucchini, egg noodles, broth, thyme, salt, and pepper to the pot.

Bring the soup to a boil, then reduce the heat to low, cover, and simmer for 8–10 minutes, or until the noodles are tender.

Adjust the seasoning as needed and bring the soup back to a simmer.

Ladle the soup into bowls and garnish with fresh parsley or cilantro, if desired.

Serve and enjoy.

Note:

You can use any type of broth that you prefer, such as vegetable or beef broth.

Add any other vegetables that you prefer, but make sure they are low in fat.

Use non-stick cooking spray in place of oil or butter to reduce the fat content.

.

Split pea and ham soup

Ingredients:

1 tablespoon oil or butter

1 onion, diced

2 cloves garlic, minced

1 cup dried green split peas, rinsed and picked through

2 cups cooked diced ham

4 cup chicken stock

1 teaspoon dried thyme

Salt and pepper to taste

1/4 cup chopped fresh parsley or cilantro (optional, for garnish)

Instructions:

Heat the oil or butter in a large pot over medium heat. Add the onion and garlic and cook until softened, about 5 minutes.

Add the split peas, ham, broth, thyme, salt, and pepper. Bring the mixture to a simmer.

Cover the pot and reduce the heat to medium-low; cook until the split peas are tender, about 45–50 minutes.

Use an immersion blender to puree some of the soup to thicken it, or puree in a blender or food processor.

Adjust the seasoning as needed and bring the soup back to a simmer.

Ladle the soup into bowls and garnish with fresh parsley or cilantro, if desired.

Serve and enjoy.

Note:

You can use other types of peas, such as yellow split peas.

Use other types of broth, such as vegetable or beef broth.

Add some cooked rice or quinoa to make it more filling.

You can also add some herbs, such as parsley, cilantro, or thyme, to add some extra flavor.

Carrot and Ginger Soup

Ingredients:

1 tablespoon oil or butter

1 onion, diced

2 cloves garlic, minced

2 cups peeled and diced carrots

1 tablespoon grated ginger

4 cups of vegetable broth

1 teaspoon ground cumin

Salt and pepper to taste

1/4 cup chopped fresh parsley or cilantro (optional, for garnish)

Instructions:

Heat the oil or butter in a large pot over medium heat. Add the onion and garlic and cook until softened, about 5 minutes.

Add the diced carrots, ginger, cumin, vegetable broth, salt, and pepper. Bring the mixture to a simmer.

Cover the pot and reduce the heat to medium-low; cook until the carrots are tender, about 20–25 minutes.

Use an immersion blender to puree the soup to a smooth consistency, or transfer the soup to a blender and puree in small batches.

Adjust the seasoning as needed and bring the soup back to a simmer.

Ladle the soup into bowls and garnish with fresh parsley or cilantro, if desired.

Serve and drink.

Note:

You can use other types of sweeteners, such as maple syrup or agave nectar.

Use other types of milk, such as soy, oat, or rice milk.

Add some cooked rice or quinoa to make it more filling.

You can also add some herbs such as parsley, cilantro, or thyme to add some extra flavor.

Carrots and ginger are a great combination of flavors, adding some sweetness and spiciness to the soup and also adding some extra fiber and potassium.

Lenten and Spinach Soup

Ingredients:

1 tablespoon oil or butter

1 onion, diced

2 cloves of garlic, minced

1 cup dried green or brown lentils, rinsed and picked through

2 cups baby spinach

4 cups of vegetable broth

1 teaspoon ground cumin

Salt and pepper to taste

1/4 cup chopped fresh parsley or cilantro (optional, for garnish)

Instructions:

Heat the oil or butter in a large pot over medium heat. Add the onion and garlic and cook until softened, about 5 minutes.

Add the lentils, spinach, broth, cumin, salt, and pepper. Bring the mixture to a simmer.

Cover the pot and reduce the heat to medium-low; cook until the lentils are tender, about 25–30 minutes.

Use an immersion blender to puree some of the soup to thicken it, or puree in a blender or food processor.

Adjust the seasoning as needed and bring the soup back to a simmer.

Ladle the soup into bowls and garnish with fresh parsley or cilantro, if desired.

Serve and enjoy.

Note:

Use other types of lentils, such as yellow or red lentils.

You can also use other types of broth, such as chicken or beef broth.

Add some cooked rice or quinoa to make it more filling.

You can also add some herbs, such as parsley, cilantro, or thyme, to add some extra flavor.

Spinach and Feta Salad

Ingredients:

6 cups fresh spinach leaves, washed and dried

1/4 cup crumbled feta cheese

1/4 cup diced red onion

1/4 cup chopped walnuts

2 tablespoons olive oil

2 tablespoons red wine vinegar

Salt and pepper to taste

Directions:

In a large bowl, combine the spinach leaves, feta cheese, red onion, and walnuts.

In a small bowl, whisk together the olive oil, red wine vinegar, salt, and pepper.

Pour the dressing over the salad and toss to combine.

Serve the salad as a healthy appetizer or side dish.

Note: Spinach and feta cheese are easy to digest, spinach is high in fiber and low in fat. Walnuts are also a good source of protein and healthy fats. Avoid high-fat options, use low-fat olive oil, and low-sodium options if possible.

Spinach and Feta Salad: This salad is packed with vitamins and minerals, and is low in fat. It can be made with fresh spinach, crumbled feta cheese, cherry tomatoes, and a simple vinaigrette made with olive oil, lemon juice, and honey.

Arugula and Quinoa Salad

This salad is high in protein and fiber, and is also low in fat. It can be made with arugula, cooked quinoa, diced tomatoes, diced cucumbers, and a simple vinaigrette made with olive oil, lemon juice, and honey.

Ingredients:

2 cups cooked quinoa, cooled

4 cups washed and dried fresh arugula leaves

1/4 cup diced red onion

1/4 cup diced red bell pepper

1/4 cup chopped fresh parsley

1/4 cup diced cucumber

2 tablespoons of olive oil

2 tablespoons fresh lemon juice

Salt and pepper to taste

Directions:

In a large bowl, combine the quinoa, arugula, red onion, red bell pepper, parsley, and cucumber.

In a small bowl, whisk together the olive oil, lemon juice, salt, and pepper.

Pour the dressing over the salad and toss to combine.

Serve the salad as a healthy appetizer or side dish.

Note: Quinoa is a good source of protein and high in fiber, and arugula is a low-calorie leafy green that is high in vitamin K and antioxidants, and it's easy to digest. Avoid high-fat options; use low-fat olive oil; and choose low-sodium options if possible.

Caesar Salad:

This classic salad is low in fat and high in protein. It can be made with romaine lettuce, croutons, and a simple dressing made with olive oil, lemon juice, and grated Parmesan cheese.

Ingredients:

1 head of Romaine lettuce, washed and dried

1/4 cup croutons (gluten-free, if desired)

1/4 cup grated Parmesan cheese

2 tablespoons of olive oil

2 tablespoons fresh lemon juice

1 clove of garlic, minced

1 teaspoon Dijon mustard

Salt and pepper to taste

Directions:

Chop the Romaine lettuce and place it in a large bowl.

Add the croutons, Parmesan cheese, olive oil, lemon juice, garlic, Dijon mustard, salt, and pepper to the bowl.

Toss the salad to combine all the ingredients.

Serve the salad as a healthy appetizer or side dish.

Note:

Romaine lettuce is high in fiber, low in fat, and easy to digest. Use low-fat options, when possible, for croutons, cheese, and olive oil. and low-sodium options if possible.

It's important to note that the traditional Caesar salad dressing contains raw egg and anchovies, which may not be suitable for some people with pancreatitis, so it's best to use a low-fat version of the dressing or make your own dressing as in the recipe above.

Greek Salad:

This salad is high in fiber and protein, and is also low in fat. It can be made with mixed greens, tomatoes, cucumbers, red onions, Kalamata olives, and feta cheese.

Ingredients:

2 cups diced tomatoes

1 cup diced cucumber

1/2 cup diced red onion

1/4 cup sliced Kalamata olives

1/4 cup crumbled feta cheese

2 tablespoons of olive oil

2 tablespoons red wine vinegar

1 teaspoon dried oregano

Salt and pepper to taste

Directions:

In a large bowl, combine the tomatoes, cucumber, red onion, Kalamata olives, and feta cheese.

In a small bowl, whisk together the olive oil, red wine vinegar, oregano, salt, and pepper.

Pour the dressing over the salad and toss to combine.

Serve the salad as a healthy appetizer or side dish.

Note: Tomatoes and cucumbers are high in water content, low in calories, and easy to digest. Feta cheese is also low in fat and easy to digest. Avoid high-fat options; use low-fat olive oil and low-sodium options if possible.

Kale and Apple Salad:

This salad is high in fiber and vitamins, and is also low in fat. It can be made with chopped kale, diced apples, toasted walnuts, and a simple vinaigrette made with olive oil, lemon juice, and honey.

Ingredients:

4 cups of kale, washed and finely chopped

2 cups of thinly sliced Granny Smith apples

1/4 cup of diced red onion

2 tablespoons of fresh lemon juice

2 tablespoons of olive oil

1/4 teaspoon of sea salt

black pepper, to taste

1/4 cup of chopped walnuts (optional)

Instructions:

In a large bowl, mix together the kale, apples, and red onion.

In a small bowl, whisk together the lemon juice, olive oil, salt, and pepper.

Drizzle the dressing over the salad and toss to combine.

If desired, top with chopped walnuts.

Serve immediately and enjoy.

Note: Kale is rich in Vitamin C and Vitamin K, which are beneficial for gut health. Additionally, apples are a good source of dietary fiber, which can help regulate bowel movements and ease constipation. However, it's best to avoid high-fat or fried food, and it's always a good idea to consult with your doctor before making any drastic changes to your diet.

Beet and Goat Cheese Salad:

This salad is high in fiber and minerals, and is also low in fat. It can be made with mixed greens, roasted beets, crumbled goat cheese, and a simple vinaigrette made with olive oil, lemon juice, and honey.

Ingredients:

3 medium-sized beets, cooked and diced

1/2 cup of crumbled goat cheese

2 tablespoons of fresh lemon juice

1 tablespoon of olive oil

1/4 teaspoon of sea salt

black pepper, to taste

1/4 cup of chopped fresh parsley or chives (optional)

Instructions:

In a large bowl, mix together the beets and crumbled goat cheese.

In a small bowl, whisk together the lemon juice, olive oil, salt, and pepper.

Drizzle the dressing over the salad and toss to combine.

If desired, top with fresh parsley or chives.

Serve immediately and enjoy.

Note: Beets are high in antioxidants, which are beneficial for gut health. Goat cheese is a good source of protein, and it's relatively low in fat compared to other cheese options. However, it's best to avoid high-fat or fried food, and it's always a good idea to consult with your doctor before making any drastic changes to your diet.

Broccoli and Cheddar Salad:

This salad is high in vitamins and protein, and is also low in fat. It can be made with broccoli florets, diced cheddar cheese, raisins, and a simple vinaigrette made with olive oil, lemon juice, and honey.

Ingredients:

4 cups of broccoli florets, blanched

1/2 cup of shredded cheddar cheese

2 tablespoons of white balsamic vinegar

1 tablespoon of olive oil

1/4 teaspoon of sea salt

Black pepper, to taste

1/4 cup of chopped fresh parsley (optional)

Instructions:

In a large bowl, mix together the broccoli florets and shredded cheddar cheese.

In a small bowl, whisk together the white balsamic vinegar, olive oil, salt, and pepper.

Drizzle the dressing over the salad and toss to combine.

If desired, top with chopped fresh parsley.

Serve immediately and enjoy.

Note: Broccoli is high in Vitamin C and Vitamin K, which are beneficial for gut health. Cheddar cheese is a good source of protein and it's relatively low in fat compared to other cheese options. However, it's best to avoid high-fat or fried food and it's always good to consult with your doctor before making any drastic changes to your diet

Cucumber and Avocado Salad:

This salad is high in fiber and healthy fats, and is also low in fat. It can be made with sliced cucumbers, diced avocados, cherry tomatoes, and a simple vinaigrette made with olive oil, lime juice, and honey.

Ingredients:

2 cups of thinly sliced cucumbers

1 avocado, peeled and diced

2 tablespoons of fresh lime juice

1 tablespoon of olive oil

1/4 teaspoon of sea salt

Black pepper, to taste

1/4 cup of chopped cilantro (optional)

Instructions:

In a large bowl, mix together the cucumbers and diced avocado.

In a small bowl, whisk together the lime juice, olive oil, salt, and pepper.

Drizzle the dressing over the salad and toss to combine.

If desired, top with chopped cilantro.

Serve immediately and enjoy.

Note: Cucumbers are high in water and antioxidants, which are beneficial for gut health. Avocado is a good source of healthy fats and fiber, which can help regulate bowel movements and ease constipation. However, it's best to avoid high-fat or fried food and it's always good to consult with your doctor before making any drastic changes to your diet.

Tomato and Mozzarella Salad:

This salad is high in vitamins and protein, and is also low in fat. It can be made with sliced tomatoes, diced mozzarella cheese, fresh basil, and a simple vinaigrette made with olive oil, balsamic vinegar, and honey.

Ingredients:

2 cups of diced tomatoes

1 cup of diced mozzarella cheese

2 tablespoons of red wine vinegar

1 tablespoon of olive oil

1/4 teaspoon of sea salt

black pepper, to taste

1/4 cup of chopped basil (optional)

Instructions:

In a large bowl, mix together the diced tomatoes and mozzarella cheese.

In a small bowl, whisk together the red wine vinegar, olive oil, salt, and pepper.

Drizzle the dressing over the salad and toss to combine.

If desired, top with chopped basil.

Serve immediately and enjoy.

Note: Tomatoes are abundant in vitamin C and vitamin K, both of which are good for intestinal health. Mozzarella cheese is high in protein and low in fat when compared to other types of cheese. However, high-fat or fried foods should be avoided, and it's always a good idea to talk with your doctor before making any major dietary changes.

Quinoa and Black Bean Salad:

This salad is high in fiber and protein, and is also low in fat. It can be made with cooked quinoa, black beans, diced tomatoes, diced cucumbers, and a simple vinaigrette made with olive oil, lime juice, and honey.

Ingredients:

1 cup cooked quinoa

1 cup cooked black beans

1/2 cup chopped red bell pepper

1/4 cup chopped red onion

2 tablespoons fresh lime juice

1 tablespoon olive oil

1/4 teaspoon sea salt

black pepper, to taste

1/4 cup chopped cilantro (optional)

Instructions:

In a large mixing bowl, combine the cooked quinoa, black beans, red bell pepper, and red onion.

In a small mixing bowl, combine the lime juice, olive oil, salt, and pepper.

Drizzle the dressing over the salad and toss to mix.

If desired, garnish with chopped cilantro.

Serve immediately and enjoy.

Quinoa is high in protein and gluten-free. Black beans are also high in dietary fiber, which can help regulate bowel motions and relieve constipation. However, it is recommended to avoid high-fat or fried foods, and it is always a good idea to talk with your doctor before making any major changes to your diet.

Healthy soups and salads might be an ideal choice for people suffering from pancreatitis. These recipes frequently include a balance of necessary elements, such as vitamins, minerals, and antioxidants, while also being low in fat and carbohydrates. Leafy greens, cruciferous vegetables, lean protein sources, and healthy fats are some examples of items that can be utilized in soups and salads for pancreatitis.

Soups made with low-fat broths or stocks, as well as veggies like broccoli, kale, and spinach, can be a healthy alternative for patients with pancreatitis. They are low in calories, high in fiber and water, and a wonderful source of vitamins and minerals.

Salads are also a wonderful option for people suffering from pancreatitis. Salads can include beets, tomatoes, cucumbers, and avocado. They are also low in calories and high in vitamins, minerals, and antioxidants, all of which are beneficial to gut health.

While soups and salads can be healthy options for people with pancreatitis, it is better to avoid high-fat or fried foods. It's also a good idea to check with your doctor before making any major dietary adjustments.

Chapter 6

Main Dishes: Meat, Fish, Poultry, and Vegetarian Options

Main meals are an important part of a well-balanced diet because they give the body the energy and nutrients it requires to function correctly. Meat, fish, poultry, and vegetarian options are all terrific choices for main courses. Each of these alternatives offers a distinct collection of nutrients and a variety of preparation methods.

Meat, such as chicken, beef, and hog, is an excellent source of protein as well as important vitamins and minerals. Fish such as salmon, tuna, and halibut are high in omega-3 fatty acids and a good source of protein. Poultry, such as turkey and duck, are lower in fat than red meats and a rich source of protein.

Beans, lentils, and tofu are other rich sources of protein and can be a nutritious alternative to meat. They are also high in dietary fiber, which can help regulate bowel motions and relieve constipation.

It is crucial to remember that for those with pancreatitis, it is preferable to choose lean cuts of meat, fish, and chicken, avoid high-fat or fried foods, and speak with a doctor before making any severe dietary changes. Additionally, it is critical to be cautious of portion sizes and to balance your main dish with a variety of veggies and fruits.

Grilled Salmon with Lemon and Herbs

Ingredients:

4 salmon fillets (about 6 ounces each)

2 tablespoons olive oil

2 tablespoons lemon juice

1 teaspoon dried thyme

1 tsp. dried rosemary

Salt and pepper, to taste

Instructions:

In a small bowl, mix together the olive oil, lemon juice, thyme, rosemary, salt, and pepper.

Place the salmon fillets in a shallow dish and pour the marinade over them, making sure they are well coated. Cover and refrigerate for at least 30 minutes.

Preheat the grill to medium-high heat.

Remove the salmon from the marinade and discard the marinade.

Grill the salmon for about 3–4 minutes per side or until the fish flakes easily with a fork.

Serve the salmon with a side of steamed vegetables or a salad for a complete and healthy meal.

Tips:

If you don't have access to a grill, you can also bake the salmon in the oven at 375°F for 12–15 minutes, or until it's cooked through.

You can also add vegetables to the skewers and grill them along with the fish for a complete and balanced meal.

This dish is high in protein and omega-3 fatty acids and low in fat. It's a great option for people with pancreatitis, as it's easy on the digestive system and provides essential nutrients. Enjoy

Baked Chicken Breast with Vegetables

132

Ingredients:

4 boneless, skinless chicken breasts

1 tablespoon olive oil

Salt and pepper, to taste

1 tbsp. dried thyme

1 tbsp. dried rosemary

2 cups of diced vegetables such as bell peppers, onions, zucchini, and carrots

1/4 cup chicken broth

Instructions:

Preheat your oven to 375°F.

In a small bowl, mix together olive oil, thyme, rosemary, salt, and pepper.

Place the chicken breasts in a baking dish and brush the mixture over the chicken.

Add the vegetables and chicken broth around the chicken.

Bake for 30–40 minutes, or until the chicken is cooked through and the vegetables are tender.

Serve with a side of whole wheat bread or a salad for a complete and healthy meal.

Tips:

You can experiment with different vegetables and seasonings to suit your taste.

If you don't have access to an oven, you can also cook this dish on the stovetop by sautéing the chicken and vegetables in a pan.

This dish is a great option for people with pancreatitis, as it's easy on the digestive system and provides essential nutrients. The baked vegetables provide a good source of fiber, vitamins, and minerals. And the chicken provides a good source of protein. Enjoy!

Turkey and Vegetable Stir-Fry

Ingredients:

1 pound of turkey breast, sliced into thin strips

1 tbsp olive oil

Salt and pepper, to taste

2 cloves of garlic, minced

1 tablespoon grated ginger

2 cups of diced vegetables such as bell peppers, onions, zucchini, and carrots

1/4 cup of chicken broth

2 tablespoons soy sauce

2 tablespoons cornstarch

Instructions:

In a small bowl, mix together soy sauce, cornstarch, and 1 tablespoon of chicken broth. Set aside.

Heat a wok or large skillet over high heat; add the olive oil. Once hot, add the turkey and stir-fry for 2–3 minutes, or until browned.

Remove the turkey from the pan and set it aside.

In the same pan, add the garlic and ginger and stir-fry for 30 seconds.

Add the diced vegetables to the pan and stir-fry for 2-3 minutes, or until they start to soften.

Add the turkey back to the pan and stir in the soy sauce mixture.

Cook for an additional 1–2 minutes or until the sauce thickens and the turkey and vegetables are evenly coated.

Serve the stir-fry over brown rice or quinoa for a complete and healthy meal.

Tips:

You can experiment with different vegetables and seasonings to suit your taste.

If you want to make this dish even healthier, use low-sodium chicken broth and soy sauce.

This dish is a great option for people with pancreatitis, as it's easy on the digestive system and provides essential nutrients. The turkey provides a good source of lean protein, and the vegetables provide a good source of fiber, vitamins, and minerals.

Grilled vegetable and tofu skewers.

Ingredients:

1 block of firm tofu, cut into 1-inch cubes

2 bell peppers, cut into 1-inch pieces

2 zucchini, cut into 1-inch slices.

1 red onion, cut into wedges

2 tablespoons olive oil

Salt and pepper, to taste

1 teaspoon dried thyme

1 teaspoon dried oregano

Skewers (soaked in water for 30 minutes before using)

Instructions:

Preheat your grill to medium-high heat.

In a small bowl, mix together olive oil, thyme, oregano, salt, and pepper.

Thread the tofu cubes, bell peppers, zucchini, and red onion onto skewers, alternating between the vegetables and tofu.

Brush the skewers with the olive oil mixture.

Grill the skewers for 8–10 minutes, turning occasionally, or until the vegetables are tender and the tofu is browned.

Serve with a side of quinoa or brown rice for a complete and healthy meal.

Tips:

You can experiment with different vegetables and seasonings to suit your taste.

If you don't have access to a grill, you can also cook these skewers in a grill pan or under a broiler.

The vegetables provide a good source of fiber, vitamins, and minerals, and tofu provides a good source of protein and calcium.

Baked Tilapia with Lemon and Herbs.

Ingredients:

4 tilapia fillets

Salt and pepper, to taste

1 lemon, thinly sliced

2 cloves of garlic, minced

2 tbsp. fresh parsley, chopped

2 tbsp. fresh thyme, chopped

2 tablespoons olive oil

Instructions:

Preheat the oven to 375 degrees F (190 degrees C).

Grease a baking dish with olive oil or line it with parchment paper.

Season the tilapia fillets with salt and pepper on both sides.

Arrange the lemon slices at the bottom of the baking dish.

Place the tilapia fillets on top of the lemon slices.

In a small bowl, mix together the garlic, parsley, thyme, and olive oil.

Brush the tilapia fillets with the olive oil mixture.

Bake the tilapia for 15-20 minutes, or until it flakes easily with a fork.

Serve the tilapia with a side of steamed vegetables or a salad for a complete and healthy meal.

Tips:

You can experiment with different herbs and seasonings to suit your taste.

If you prefer a stronger lemon flavor, you can squeeze some fresh lemon juice over the fish before baking.

Tilapia is a lean fish, low in fat and calories but high in protein, vitamins, and minerals. The lemon, herbs, and olive oil give the fish a bright, flavorful taste, and the fish is cooked with the skin on, which helps to keep the fish moist during cooking.

Vegetable and Bean Enchiladas.

Ingredients:

1 tbsp vegetable oil

1 onion, diced

1 red bell pepper, diced

1 yellow bell pepper, diced

1 zucchini, diced

1 can of black beans, rinsed and drained

1/2 teaspoon cumin

Salt and pepper, to taste

1 cup of enchilada sauce

8 whole wheat tortillas

1 cup of shredded cheese (cheddar or Monterey jack)

Chop fresh cilantro for garnish.

Instructions:

Preheat your oven to 375 degrees F (190 degrees C).

Heat the vegetable oil in a large skillet over medium heat. Add the onion, bell peppers, and zucchini. Cook, stirring occasionally, until the vegetables are tender, about 10 minutes.

Stir in the black beans, cumin, salt, and pepper. Cook for 2 minutes more.

Spread 1/4 cup of enchilada sauce over the bottom of a 9-by-13-inch baking dish.

Spread about 1/2 cup of the vegetable mixture over each tortilla. Roll up the tortillas and place them seam-side down in the baking dish.

Pour the remaining enchilada sauce over the top of the enchiladas and sprinkle with shredded cheese.

Cover the baking dish with aluminum foil and bake for 20 minutes. Remove the foil and bake for an additional 10 minutes or until the cheese is melted and bubbly.

Let the enchiladas cool for 5 minutes before serving. Garnish with cilantro.

Tips:

You can experiment with different vegetables, beans, and sauces to suit your taste.

This recipe is also very flexible; you can add some chicken, pork, or beef if you desire.

You can use store-bought or homemade enchilada sauce; just make sure it's low in sodium.

Slow Cooker Chicken and Vegetable Stew.

Ingredients:

1 pound boneless, skinless chicken breasts, cut into bite-size pieces.

2 cups potatoes, diced

1 cup diced carrots

1 cup diced celery

1 onion, diced

2 cloves of garlic, minced

1 cup chicken broth (low-sodium)

1 cup of water

2 teaspoon dried thyme

1 tsp. dried rosemary

Salt and pepper, to taste

2 tablespoons cornstarch

2 tablespoons water

Instructions:

In a slow cooker, combine chicken, potatoes, carrots, celery, onion, garlic, chicken broth, water, thyme, rosemary, salt, and pepper.

Cook on low heat for 6–8 hours or on high heat for 3–4 hours, until the chicken is cooked through and the vegetables are tender.

In a small bowl, mix the cornstarch and 2 tablespoons of water together. Stir the mixture into the slow cooker.

Cook on high heat for an additional 30 minutes, or until the stew has thickened.

Serve hot and enjoy.

Tips:

You can use any vegetables you have on hand, such as turnips, parsnips, or sweet potatoes.

To make this recipe vegetarian, omit the chicken and use vegetable broth instead of chicken broth.

If you want to thicken the stew more, you can add more cornstarch mixture or mash some of the vegetables.

This dish is a great option for people with pancreatitis, as it is a low-fat, high-fiber, nutrient-dense meal that is easy to digest. The slow cooker makes it convenient and easy to prepare, and it's a great way to use up any vegetables you have in your fridge.

Lentil and Vegetable Curry.

Ingredients:

1 cup dried green or brown lentils, rinsed and drained

2 cups of water

1 tablespoon olive oil

1 onion, diced

2 cloves of garlic, minced

1 teaspoon ground cumin

1 teaspoon ground coriander

1 teaspoon ground turmeric

1/2 teaspoon ground ginger

1/2 teaspoon ground cinnamon

1/4 teaspoon cayenne pepper (optional)

2 cups diced vegetables of your choice (such as carrots, bell peppers, zucchini, etc.)

1 can of diced tomatoes (14.5 oz)

1 cup vegetable broth (low-sodium)

Salt and pepper, to taste

1/4 cup fresh cilantro, chopped (optional)

1/4 cup plain yogurt or sour cream (optional)

Instructions:

In a medium saucepan, bring the lentils and water to a boil. Reduce the heat to low and simmer for 20–25 minutes, or until the lentils are tender. Drain and set aside any excess water.

In a large skillet or pot, heat the olive oil over medium heat. Add the onion and garlic and cook for 3–4 minutes, or until softened.

Add the cumin, coriander, turmeric, ginger, cinnamon, and cayenne pepper (if using) and cook for 1-2 minutes, or until fragrant.

Add the diced vegetables and cook for 5-7 minutes, or until they are tender.

Stir in the diced tomatoes, vegetable broth, and cooked lentils. Bring to a boil, then reduce the heat to low and let it simmer for 10–15 minutes, or until the vegetables are tender and the sauce has thickened.

Season with salt and pepper to taste.

Serve hot, topped with fresh cilantro and yogurt or sour cream, if desired.

Tips:

You can use any vegetables you have on hand and any kind of lentils you prefer.

You can also add some protein of your choice, like chicken, shrimp, or tofu.

This dish can be served with rice, quinoa, or naan bread.

This dish is a great option for people with pancreatitis, as it is a low-fat, high-fiber, nutrient-dense meal that is easy to digest. Lentils are a great source of protein, and the vegetables and spices used in this dish provide a variety of vitamins and minerals. The curry can be easily customized to suit your taste and dietary needs, and it's a great way to use up any vegetables you have in your fridge.

Quinoa and Black Bean Burrito Bowls.

Ingredients:

1 cup quinoa, rinsed and drained

2 cups of water

1 tablespoon olive oil

1 onion, diced

2 cloves of garlic, minced

1 teaspoon ground cumin

1 teaspoon chili powder

1/2 teaspoon ground coriander

1 can of black beans (14.5 oz), rinsed and drained

1 cup diced tomatoes

1/2 cup corn kernels

1/4 cup fresh cilantro, chopped

Salt and pepper, to taste

Toppings:

Shredded lettuce

Diced avocado

Shredded cheddar cheese

Sour cream or plain yogurt

Salsa

Instructions:

In a medium saucepan, bring the quinoa and water to a boil. Reduce the heat to low and simmer for 20–25 minutes, or until the quinoa is cooked and the water has been absorbed.

While the quinoa is cooking, heat the olive oil in a large skillet over medium heat. Add the onion and garlic and cook for 3–4 minutes, or until softened.

Add the cumin, chili powder, and coriander and cook for 1-2 minutes, or until fragrant.

Stir in the black beans, diced tomatoes, and corn kernels. Cook for 5–7 minutes, or until the vegetables are tender.

Stir in the cooked quinoa and fresh cilantro. Season with salt and pepper to taste.

Serve the quinoa and black bean mixture in bowls and top with shredded lettuce, diced avocado, shredded cheddar cheese, sour cream or yogurt, and salsa.

Tips:

You can also add some protein of your choice, like chicken, shrimp, or tofu.

This dish can be served with brown rice or lettuce leaves as a wrap.

This dish is a great option for people with pancreatitis, as it is a low-fat, high-fiber, nutrient-dense meal that is easy to digest. Quinoa is a great source of protein, and black beans are a great source of fiber, and the spices and vegetables used in this dish provide a variety of vitamins and minerals. The burrito bowl can be easily customized to suit your taste and dietary needs, and it's a great way to use up any vegetables or beans you have in your fridge.

Stuffed Portobello Mushrooms.

Ingredients:

4 large Portobello mushroom caps

1 tablespoon of olive oil

1/2 cup diced onion

1/2 cup diced bell pepper

2 cloves of garlic, minced

1/2 cup cooked quinoa

1/2 cup diced tomatoes

1/4 cup chopped fresh parsley

1/4 cup grated Parmesan cheese

Salt and pepper to taste

Directions:

Preheat the oven to 350°F.

Clean the mushroom caps and remove the stems.

In a pan, heat olive oil over medium heat. Add onion, bell pepper, and garlic, and sauté until softened.

Stir in the cooked quinoa, diced tomatoes, parsley, parmesan cheese, salt, and pepper.

Spoon the mixture into the mushroom caps, filling them evenly.

Place the mushrooms on a baking sheet and bake for 20–25 minutes, or until the mushrooms are tender and the filling is heated through.

Serve hot and enjoy.

Optional: You can top with more grated Parmesan cheese or bread crumbs before baking for added texture.

In conclusion, main courses are an important part of any meal, and there are numerous selections available, including meat, fish, poultry, and vegetarian options. Meat meals can include steak, pork, and lamb, which are frequently cooked using methods such as grilling, roasting, or braising. Fish and seafood dishes are high in lean protein and can be prepared in a variety of ways, such as grilling, sautéing, or baking.

Poultry meals, such as chicken and turkey, can be prepared in a similar manner and are typically considered a healthier alternative to red meats. Vegetarian alternatives include foods prepared with plant-based proteins such as tofu, tempeh, and seitan, as well as dishes made with vegetables and grains such as quinoa, lentils, and rice.

Each of these options has its own distinct flavor and nutritional benefits, and there are numerous recipes and preparation methods to select from. When choosing the correct main dish for a dinner, it is critical to consider one's dietary limitations, tastes, and health goals.

CHAPTER 7

Side Dishes and Vegetable Recipes for Pancreatitis.

Pancreatitis is a condition in which the pancreas, an organ responsible for producing enzymes that aid digestion, becomes inflamed. This can result in a variety of symptoms, such as abdominal pain, nausea, and vomiting. Pancreatitis patients are frequently advised to follow a special diet to reduce the strain on the pancreas. One important aspect of this diet is the inclusion of a variety of nutrient-dense side dishes and vegetable recipes.

Side dishes and vegetable recipes can provide important vitamins, minerals, and antioxidants that are necessary for overall health. They're also a great way to get more fiber into your diet, which can help regulate digestion and keep your gut healthy. Vegetables high in vitamins and minerals, such as leafy greens, broccoli, bell peppers, and sweet potatoes, are excellent choices for those with pancreatitis. Additionally, high-fat, high-sugar, and spicy foods should be avoided as they can aggravate symptoms.

Roasted vegetables, steamed green beans or asparagus, sautéed spinach, and a mixed green salad with a simple vinaigrette dressing are some suitable side dishes and vegetable recipes for those with pancreatitis. These can be prepared with a few oils and seasonings to reduce pancreatic stress and provide maximum health benefits.

Roasted Vegetables.

Ingredients:

2 bell peppers, seeded and cut into chunks

2 zucchini, cut into chunks.

2 sweet potatoes, peeled and cut into chunks

1 onion, cut into wedges

2 cloves of garlic, minced

2 tablespoons of olive oil

1 teaspoon dried oregano

1/2 teaspoon dried thyme

Salt and pepper to taste

Directions:

Preheat the oven to 400°F.

In a large bowl, combine the bell peppers, zucchinis, sweet potatoes, onions, and garlic.

Add the olive oil, oregano, thyme, salt, and pepper, and toss to coat the vegetables evenly.

Spread the vegetables out in a single layer on a baking sheet.

Roast for 25–30 minutes, or until the vegetables are tender and slightly golden brown, stirring occasionally.

Serve hot as a side dish or toss with quinoa or pasta for a main dish.

Optional: You can add other vegetables like broccoli, cauliflower, and mushrooms to this recipe to make it more colorful and flavorful.

Steamed Green Beans.

Ingredients:

1 pound fresh green beans, trimmed ends

1 tablespoon butter or olive oil

1 clove of garlic, minced (optional)

Salt and pepper to taste

Lemon juice (optional)

Directions:

Fill a large pot with about an inch of water and bring to a boil over high heat.

Place a steamer basket in the pot, and add the green beans to the basket.

Cover the pot with a lid and steam the green beans for about 5 minutes, or until tender.

While the green beans are steaming, melt the butter or heat the olive oil in a small pan over medium heat.

Add the minced garlic and cook for 1-2 minutes, or until fragrant.

Remove the green beans from the steamer basket and place them in a serving dish.

Pour the butter or oil and garlic over the green beans and toss to coat.

Season with salt and pepper to taste.

Serve hot with a squeeze of lemon juice over the top, if desired.

Optional: You can add other herbs like parsley, thyme, or basil to the butter or oil, or you can sprinkle with toasted almonds or cashews for added crunch.

Sautéed Spinach

Ingredients:

2 tablespoons of olive oil

2 cloves of garlic, minced

1 pound of fresh spinach leaves, washed and dried

Salt and pepper to taste

Lemon juice (optional)

Directions:

Heat the olive oil in a large skillet over medium heat.

Add the minced garlic and cook for 1-2 minutes, or until fragrant.

Add the spinach leaves to the skillet and stir to coat with the oil and garlic.

Cook for 2–3 minutes, or until the spinach is wilted and tender.

Season with salt and pepper to taste.

Serve hot with a squeeze of lemon juice over the top, if desired.

Optional: You can add some nuts like pine nuts, walnuts, or slivered almonds to the skillet for added crunch and flavor. You can also add some red pepper flakes for a spicy kick.

Mixed Green Salad.

Ingredients:

4 cups mixed greens (such as lettuce, arugula, and spinach)

1/4 cup cherry tomatoes, halved

1/4 cup diced cucumber

1/4 cup diced red onion

1/4 cup peeled and diced jicama

1/4 cup crumbled low-fat cheese (optional)

For the vinaigrette:

2 tablespoons of olive oil

1 tablespoon apple cider vinegar

1 teaspoon Dijon mustard

1/4 teaspoon honey

Salt and pepper to taste

Directions:

In a large bowl, combine the mixed greens, cherry tomatoes, cucumber, red onion, jicama, and cheese (if using).

In a small bowl, whisk together the olive oil, apple cider vinegar, Dijon mustard, honey, salt, and pepper.

Drizzle the vinaigrette over the salad and toss to coat the greens evenly.

Serve immediately and enjoy the freshness of the salad.

Note: Individuals with pancreatitis should avoid high-fat foods, so it is best to use low-fat cheese and oil. Also, it's important to avoid high-fat dressings like Ranch or Thousand Island, so vinaigrette is a great option as it's low in fat and high in flavor. Additionally, jicama is a great addition as it is a low-calorie, low-carb, and low-fat vegetable that provides a good source of dietary fiber.

Grilled Eggplant.

Ingredients:

1 large eggplant, sliced into 1/2-inch thick rounds

2 tablespoons of olive oil

Salt and pepper to taste

1/4 cup chopped fresh basil leaves

1/4 cup chopped fresh mint leaves

2 cloves of garlic, minced

2 tablespoons balsamic vinegar

2 tablespoons of lemon juice

Directions:

Preheat the grill to medium-high heat.

Brush the eggplant slices with olive oil and season with salt and pepper.

Grill the eggplant for about 3–4 minutes per side, or until tender and slightly charred.

While the eggplant is grilling, in a small bowl, mix together the basil, mint, garlic, balsamic vinegar, and lemon juice.

Once the eggplant is done grilling, remove it from the grill and place it on a serving platter.

Drizzle the herb mixture over the eggplant.

Serve as a side dish, or top with a sprinkle of low-fat cheese and serve as a main dish.

Note: Eggplant is a good source of dietary fiber and low in calories and fats, making it a great option for individuals with pancreatitis. Additionally, the balsamic vinegar and lemon juice in the herb mixture provide a nice balance of flavor without adding too much fat.

Baked Squash.

Ingredients:

1 medium-sized acorn or butternut squash, peeled and cut into 1-inch cubes

2 tablespoons of olive oil

Salt and pepper to taste

1 teaspoon ground cinnamon (optional)

1 teaspoon ground nutmeg (optional)

2 tablespoons maple syrup or honey

2 tablespoons chopped fresh herbs (such as thyme, rosemary, or sage) (optional)

Directions:

Preheat the oven to 375°F (190°C).

In a large mixing bowl, toss the squash cubes with the olive oil, salt, pepper, cinnamon, and nutmeg (if using) until they are evenly coated.

Spread the squash cubes in a single layer on a baking sheet lined with parchment paper.

Drizzle the maple syrup or honey over the squash cubes.

Bake for 25–30 minutes, or until the squash is tender and lightly browned.

Remove the squash from the oven and toss with fresh herbs (if using).

Serve as a side dish or add some cooked lean protein like chicken or fish to make it a main dish.

Note: Squash is a good source of dietary fiber and low in calories and fats making it a great option for individuals with pancreatitis. Additionally, the maple syrup or honey provides a nice balance of flavor without adding too much fat.

Broccoli and cauliflower.

Ingredients:

1 head of broccoli, cut into florets

1 head of cauliflower, cut into florets

2 tablespoons of olive oil

Salt and pepper to taste

2 cloves of garlic, minced

2 tablespoons of lemon juice

2 tablespoons grated Parmesan cheese (optional)

Directions:

Preheat the oven to 400°F (200°C).

In a large mixing bowl, toss the broccoli and cauliflower florets with olive oil, salt, pepper, and minced garlic.

Spread the vegetables in a single layer on a baking sheet lined with parchment paper.

Roast for 15-20 minutes, or until the vegetables are tender and lightly browned.

Remove the vegetables from the oven and toss with lemon juice.

Serve as a side dish or add some cooked lean protein like chicken or fish to make it a main dish.

Optionally, you can also add some grated Parmesan cheese on top just before serving for a cheesy touch.

Note: The lemon juice provides a nice balance of flavor without adding too much fat.

Grilled Zucchini.

Ingredients:

2 medium zucchini, sliced about 1/4 inch thick lengthwise.

2 tablespoons of olive oil

Season with salt and pepper to taste.

1 tablespoon fresh basil, chopped (optional)

Directions:

Preheat the grill to a medium-high temperature.

Toss the zucchini slices with the olive oil, salt, and pepper in a large mixing bowl.

Grill the zucchini slices for approximately 2–3 minutes per side, or until grill marks emerge and the zucchini is soft.

Take off the grill and stir in the fresh basil (if using).

Serve right away.

As with the last meal, it is vital to avoid high-fat and high-sugar items when on a pancreatitis diet, so substituting olive oil for butter or other fats is a wise alternative. Grilled zucchini is a wonderful and healthful way to reap the benefits of this vegetable without adding any additional substances that may be damaging to the pancreas.

Roasted Carrots.

Ingredients:

1 oz. of carrots, peeled and cut into 2-inch pieces.

2 tablespoons of olive oil

Salt and pepper, to taste

1 tablespoon chopped fresh thyme (optional)

Directions:

Preheat the oven to 400 degrees F (200 degrees C).

In a large mixing bowl, toss the carrots with olive oil, salt, and pepper.

Spread the carrots out in a single layer on a baking sheet.

Roast in the preheated oven for 20–25 minutes, or until the carrots are tender and lightly browned.

Remove from the oven and toss with fresh thyme (if using).

Serve immediately.

Note: Using olive oil instead of butter or other fats is a good choice. Also, this recipe is a simple way to enjoy the benefits of carrots without adding any additional ingredients that may be harmful to the pancreas.

Grilled Peppers.

Ingredients:

2 red, yellow, or green bell peppers, cut into 2-inch chunks.

2 tablespoons of olive oil

Season with salt and pepper to taste.

1 teaspoon minced garlic (optional)

Directions:

Preheat the grill to a medium-high temperature.

Toss the bell pepper slices with the olive oil, salt, and pepper in a large mixing bowl.

Grill the bell pepper slices for 5-7 minutes per side, or until grill marks form and the peppers are soft.

Remove from the grill and mix with garlic powder (if using)

Serve right away.

As with the preceding meals, it is crucial to avoid high-fat and high-sugar items when following a pancreatitis diet, so substituting olive oil for butter or other fats is a smart option. Grilled bell peppers are a wonderful and healthful way to reap the benefits of this vegetable without adding any additional additives that may be damaging to the pancreas.

Note: It is important to consult with a healthcare professional or a dietitian before making any significant changes to your diet, especially if you have a medical condition.

Finally, when following a pancreatitis diet, it is critical to restrict high-fat and high-sugar items.

Roasting or grilling vegetables like carrots, zucchini, and bell peppers is an easy and healthful way to get their advantages without adding any additional chemicals that may be damaging to the pancreas.

These side dishes are simple to create, and the addition of olive oil, salt, pepper, and fresh herbs such as thyme and basil can improve the flavor and make them wonderful. These recipes can be used as a reference to make other simple and healthy pancreatitis-friendly vegetable dishes.

CHAPTER 8

Healthy Snacks and Desserts for Pancreatitis

When following a pancreatitis diet, it is critical to avoid high-fat and high-sugar foods. This can make it difficult to find nutritious and filling snacks and sweets. However, there are numerous options that are not only tasty but also beneficial to maintaining a healthy pancreas.

Fresh fruits and vegetables, as well as low-fat dairy products like yogurt and cheese, are examples of nutritious snacks. Desserts can be made healthier by adding natural sweeteners like honey or maple syrup, as well as whole grains and alternative flours like almond flour.

It's also vital to watch portion sizes and keep track of your entire daily calorie intake. Fruit sorbet, fresh fruit smoothies, yogurt parfaits, baked apple slices with cinnamon, and homemade granola bars are all good for a pancreatitis diet. These selections are not only delicious, but they also include important nutrients and can help maintain a healthy pancreas.

Overall, the key to a healthy pancreatitis diet is to eat nutrient-dense foods, restrict processed foods and added sweets, and keep track of portion sizes.

Fresh fruit salad

Ingredients:

2 cups mixed berries (strawberries, blueberries, raspberries, and blackberries)

1 large peeled and chopped mango

2 medium peeled and sliced kiwis

2 medium peeled and segmented oranges

1/2 cup seedless grapes, cut in half

two tablespoons of honey

1 tbsp. freshly squeezed lemon juice

Directions:

Combine the mixed berries, diced mango, sliced kiwi, orange segments, and split grapes in a large mixing bowl.

In a small mixing bowl, combine the honey and lemon juice.

Gently mix the fruit in the honey-lemon dressing to coat.

Refrigerate for at least 30 minutes to let the flavors combine.

Enjoy while it's cold!

Note: This dish is a terrific way to enjoy a variety of fruits and may be customized to your liking. You can substitute different fruits or utilize seasonal fruits. The honey and lemon dressing can also be tailored to your preferences.

This recipe is ideal for a healthy and refreshing snack or dessert for individuals on a pancreatitis diet because it contains natural sweeteners and is low in fat.

Greek yogurt with honey and mixed berries.

Ingredients:

1 cup Greek yogurt, plain

1 cup mixed berries (strawberries, blueberries, raspberries, and blackberries)

two tablespoons of honey

1 tablespoon vanilla extract

1/4 teaspoon cinnamon powder (optional)

Directions:

Combine the Greek yogurt, vanilla essence, and ground cinnamon in a medium mixing bowl (if using).

Heat the mixed berries and honey in a small saucepan over medium heat until the berries soften and release their juices.

Remove from the heat and set aside to cool for a few minutes.

Top the yogurt mixture with the heated berry mixture in a serving bowl.

Serve and have fun!

Greek yogurt is high in protein, while the mixed berries and honey give it natural sweetness. Because it contains natural sweeteners and is low in fat, this recipe is ideal for a healthy and tasty snack or dessert for individuals on a pancreatitis diet.

Use any type of berry you choose, or you can use frozen berries if fresh berries aren't in season. You can also tailor the amount of honey to your preferences.

Thinly sliced sweet potatoes.

Ingredients:

2 medium peeled and thinly sliced sweet potatoes

2 teaspoons of olive oil

a quarter teaspoon of salt

a quarter teaspoon of black pepper

1/4 teaspoon cinnamon powder

Directions:

Preheat the oven to 400 degrees Fahrenheit (200 degrees Celsius). Line a baking sheet with parchment paper.

Toss the sweet potato slices with olive oil, salt, black pepper, and ground cinnamon in a large mixing bowl.

On the prepared baking sheet, arrange the sweet potato slices in a single layer.

Bake for 20–25 minutes, or until the chips are golden brown and crispy, flipping halfway through.

Remove from the oven and set aside for a few minutes to cool before serving.

Sweet potato chips are a tasty and healthy alternative to ordinary potato chips. They are abundant in fiber and vitamins while being low in fat. Because it is low in fat and contains no added sugar, this meal is an excellent choice for a healthy and enjoyable snack for individuals on a pancreatitis diet. Seasonings can be changed to your liking; experiment with other herbs or spices to spice things up. You can also use other root vegetables, like beets or parsnips, in this recipe.

Apple slices with almond butter.

Ingredients:

2 medium apples, cored and sliced

1/4 cup of almond butter

1 tablespoon of honey (optional)

1 teaspoon of cinnamon (optional)

Directions:

In a small bowl, mix together the almond butter and honey (if using) until smooth.

Spread the almond butter mixture over the apple slices and sprinkle with cinnamon (if using).

Serve immediately and enjoy as a healthy and satisfying snack.

Note: This recipe is a perfect option for a healthy and satisfying snack for those following a diet for pancreatitis, as it is low in fat and doesn't use any added sugar. Apples are a good source of fiber and vitamins, while almond butter is a good source of healthy fats and protein.

Add some nuts or seeds to this recipe to make it more nutritious and filling. You can also try this recipe with other fruits such as pears, bananas, or peaches.

Carrot sticks with hummus.

Ingredients:

1 pound of carrots, peeled and cut into sticks

1 cup of hummus

1 tablespoon of lemon juice (optional)

1/4 teaspoon of cumin (optional)

Salt and pepper to taste

Directions:

In a medium mixing bowl, combine the hummus, lemon juice (if using), cumin (if using), salt, and pepper. Mix until well combined.

Serve the hummus on a plate or in a bowl, and arrange the carrot sticks on the side.

Serve and enjoy as a healthy and satisfying snack.

Note: Carrots are a good source of fiber and vitamins, while hummus is a good source of protein and healthy fats. This recipe is a perfect option for a healthy and satisfying snack for those following a diet for pancreatitis, as it is low in fat and doesn't use any added sugar.

You can also try this recipe with other vegetables such as celery, bell peppers, or cucumbers. You can also adjust the seasoning to your liking and make your own hummus or use store-bought.

Quinoa and black bean salad.

Ingredients:

1 cup of quinoa, rinsed and drained

1 can of black beans, drained and rinsed

1 red bell pepper, diced

1/2 red onion, diced

1 jalapeno pepper, seeded and diced (optional)

2 cloves of garlic, minced

2 tablespoons of olive oil

2 tablespoons of fresh lime juice

1 teaspoon of ground cumin

Salt and pepper to taste

Fresh cilantro or parsley, chopped (optional)

Directions:

In a medium saucepan, bring 2 cups of water to a boil. Add the quinoa and reduce the heat to low. Cover and simmer for 18–20 minutes, or until the quinoa is tender and the water is absorbed. Remove from the heat and set aside to cool.

In a large mixing bowl, combine the quinoa, black beans, red bell pepper, red onion, jalapeno pepper (if using), and garlic.

In a small mixing bowl, whisk together the olive oil, lime juice, cumin, salt, and pepper. Pour the dressing over the salad and toss to combine.

Refrigerate for at least 30 minutes to allow the flavors to meld together.

Before serving, garnish with fresh cilantro or parsley (if using) and toss again.

Serve and enjoy this healthy and satisfying salad.

Note: Quinoa is a protein-rich grain, while black beans are a good source of protein and fiber. This recipe is a perfect option for a healthy and satisfying meal for those following a diet for pancreatitis, as it is low in fat and doesn't use any added sugar.

You can adjust the seasoning and the vegetables to your liking. You can also add some avocado, corn, or tomatoes to this recipe to make it more nutritious and filling. You can also use this recipe as a side dish or as a main dish.

Chia seed pudding.

Ingredients:

1/2 cup of chia seeds

2 cups of almond milk (or other non-dairy milk)

1/4 cup of honey or maple syrup (or sweetener of choice)

1 teaspoon of vanilla extract

1/4 teaspoon of ground cinnamon (optional)

A pinch of salt

Fresh fruit, nuts, or coconut flakes for topping (optional)

Directions:

In a medium mixing bowl, combine the chia seeds, almond milk, honey, vanilla extract, cinnamon (if using), and salt. Whisk until well combined.

Cover the bowl with plastic wrap and refrigerate for at least 2 hours or overnight.

Before serving, give the pudding a good stir and then divide it into serving cups or bowls.

If desired, top each serving with fresh fruit, nuts, or coconut flakes.

Serve and enjoy as a healthy and satisfying dessert.

Note: Chia seeds are a good source of fiber, protein, and healthy fats. This recipe is a perfect option for a healthy and satisfying dessert for those following a diet for pancreatitis, as it is low in fat and doesn't use any added sugar. The sweetener can be adjusted to your liking and also try different flavors like cocoa powder, peanut butter, or matcha powder.

You can also use different types of milk or yogurt. It can be prepared in advance and enjoy it during the week as a healthy snack or breakfast.

Frozen yogurt bark.

Ingredients:

2 cups of plain Greek yogurt

1/4 cup of honey or maple syrup (or sweetener of choice)

1 teaspoon of vanilla extract

1/2 cup of fresh berries, chopped

1/4 cup of chopped nuts, such as almonds or pistachios (optional)

Directions:

Line a baking sheet with parchment paper or a silicone mat.

In a large mixing bowl, combine the Greek yogurt, honey, and vanilla extract. Whisk until well combined.

Fold in the fresh berries and chopped nuts (if using) until evenly distributed.

Spread the yogurt mixture onto the prepared baking sheet, using a spatula to create an even layer.

Freeze for at least 2 hours, or until solid.

Once frozen, remove the bark from the baking sheet by lifting the edges of the parchment paper or silicone mat. Break it into bite-sized pieces.

Keep the bark in an airtight container in the freezer.

Before serving, remove the bark from the freezer for about 5–10 minutes to soften.

Serve and enjoy as a healthy and satisfying frozen dessert.

Note: Greek yogurt is a good source of protein and probiotics. This recipe is a perfect option for a frozen dessert for those following a diet for pancreatitis, as it is low in fat and doesn't use any added sugar. You can change the sweetener to your liking and also try different flavors and toppings like chocolate chips, coconut flakes, or granola.

Different types of yogurt, can be used. You can also prepare it in advance and enjoy it whenever you want as a healthy snack or dessert.

Apple slices baked with cinnamon.

Ingredients:

3 medium-sized apples, cored and sliced

1 tablespoon of lemon juice

1 teaspoon of ground cinnamon

1/4 teaspoon of nutmeg

2 tablespoons of honey or maple syrup (or sweetener of choice)

A pinch of salt

Directions:

Preheat the oven to 350°F (175°C). Line a baking sheet with parchment paper or a silicone mat.

In a medium mixing bowl, combine the apple slices, lemon juice, cinnamon, nutmeg, honey, and salt. Toss until the apple slices are evenly coated.

Arrange the apple slices on the prepared baking sheet in a single layer.

Bake for 20–25 minutes, or until the apples are tender and lightly caramelized.

Allow to cool for a few minutes before serving after removing from the oven.

serve as a healthy and satisfying snack or dessert.

Note: Apples are a good source of fiber and vitamin C. This recipe is a perfect option for a healthy and satisfying snack or dessert for those following a diet for pancreatitis, as it is low in fat and doesn't use any added sugar.

Adjust the sweetener to your liking and also try different spices like ginger, allspice, or cardamom. You can also use different types of sweetener, like agave syrup or brown sugar. Prepare it in advance and enjoy it during the week as a healthy snack or breakfast.

Homemade granola bars.

Ingredients:

2 cups of rolled oats

1/2 cup of chopped nuts, such as almonds, walnuts, or pecans

1/2 cup of dried fruit, such as cranberries, raisins, or chopped apricots

1/4 cup of sunflower seeds

1/4 cup of pumpkin seeds

1/4 cup of chia seeds

1/4 cup of flax seeds

1/4 cup of honey or maple syrup

1/4 cup of coconut oil

1 teaspoon of vanilla extract

A pinch of salt

Directions:

Preheat the oven to 350°F (175°C). Line an 8-by-8-inch baking pan with parchment paper or a silicone mat.

In a large mixing bowl, combine the oats, nuts, dried fruit, sunflower seeds, pumpkin seeds, chia seeds, flax seeds, honey, coconut oil, vanilla extract, and salt. Mix until well combined.

Press the mixture into the prepared baking pan using a spatula or your hands to create an even layer.

Bake for 20–25 minutes, or until the granola bars are golden brown and fragrant.

Remove from the oven and set aside for 30 minutes before cutting into bars.

serve as a healthy and satisfying snack or breakfast.

Note: This recipe is a perfect diet for pancreatitis, as it is low in fat, high in protein and fiber, and doesn't use any added sugar. You can adjust the sweetener to your liking and also try different ingredients like chocolate chips, coconut flakes, or different types of nuts.

Use different types of sweetener, like agave syrup or brown sugar. You can also prepare it in advance and enjoy it during the week as a healthy snack or breakfast.

To conclude, it is critical to focus on foods that are low in fat, high in fiber and protein, and easy to digest when following a pancreatitis diet. Healthy snacks and desserts can fulfill your desires while also supplying important nutrients.

Fresh fruit salad, Greek yogurt with honey and mixed berries, thinly sliced sweet potatoes lightly fried in olive oil and seasoned with salt, pepper, and cinnamon, apple slices with almond butter, carrot sticks with hummus, quinoa and black bean salad, chia seed pudding, frozen yogurt bark, apple slices baked with cinnamon, and homemade granola bars are just a few of the options. All of these options are simple to prepare and may be tailored to your preferences and dietary requirements. Always speak with your healthcare provider before making any dietary adjustments.

CHAPTER 9

Beverages: Juices, Smoothies, and Teas for Pancreatitis.

Beverages can be a significant part of a pancreatitis diet. They can supply hydration, nutrients, and even aid in digestion. Choosing the correct sorts of beverages to maintain a healthy pancreas is critical. Juices, smoothies, and teas can all be beneficial for those suffering from pancreatitis, but it's critical to be aware of the ingredients and preparation techniques.

Drinks are an excellent source of vitamins and minerals, but it is critical to select juices that are low in sugar and high in fiber. Freshly squeezed fruits and vegetables are the finest options, but restrict your fruit juice consumption because it might be heavy in sugar.

Smoothies are an easy way to incorporate a variety of fruits and vegetables into your diet. They are easily customizable to your preferences and dietary requirements. To balance out the smoothie, pick low-sugar fruits and add healthy fats and proteins.

Teas can help with digestion and give hydration to people suffering from pancreatitis. Herbal teas, such as ginger, peppermint, and chamomile, can be especially good for people suffering from pancreatitis. Caffeine-containing teas should be avoided since they can irritate the pancreas.

When it comes to beverages and pancreatitis, the idea is to find low-sugar, high-nutrient ones. It's also vital to be cautious of the ingredients and methods of preparation and to always speak with your healthcare professional before making any dietary adjustments.

Freshly squeezed carrot and ginger juice.

Ingredients:

1 lb. carrots, peeled and chopped

2 inch piece of peeled and chopped ginger

1/2 lemon, juiced

2 tbsp. honey (optional)

Instructions:

Run the carrots and ginger through a juicer.

Stir in the lemon juice and honey (if using).

Taste and adjust sweetness or acidity as desired.

Serve immediately and enjoy!

Note: You can also use a blender to make the juice; in that case, you will have to strain the juice before serving.

Green smoothie.

Ingredients:

1 cup fresh spinach

1 cup of fresh kale

1/2 avocado

1/2 banana

1/2 cup fresh pineapple

1/2 cup fresh cucumber

1/2 cup unsweetened almond milk

1/2 cup filtered water

1/2 teaspoon ginger powder

Instructions:

Rinse the spinach, kale, avocado, banana, pineapple, and cucumber.

Cut the avocado and banana into chunks.

In a blender, combine the spinach, kale, avocado, banana, pineapple, cucumber, almond milk, water, and ginger powder.

Blend on high speed until smooth and creamy.

Taste and adjust seasonings as needed.

Pour the smoothie into a glass and enjoy it immediately.

Note:

It's recommended to consult with a healthcare professional before adding ginger powder if you have pancreatitis.

It's also important to consume the smoothie in moderation and not as a replacement for a well-rounded diet.

If you're experiencing a flare-up of pancreatitis, it may be best to avoid high-fat foods like avocado and stick to lower-fat options like cucumber and spinach.

Apple, beet, and ginger juice.

Ingredients:

2 medium apples

1 medium beet

1 inch of ginger

1/2 cup filtered water

Instructions:

Rinse the apples, beets, and ginger.

Cut the apples and beets into chunks.

Peel the ginger using a spoon or a peeler.

In a juicer, juice the apples, beets, ginger, and filtered water.

Stir the juice well and taste for seasoning; adjust as needed.

Pour the juice into a glass and enjoy it immediately.

Note:

It's recommended to consult with a healthcare professional before adding ginger if you have pancreatitis.

It's also important to consume the juice in moderation and not as a replacement for a well-rounded diet.

If you're experiencing a flare-up of pancreatitis, it may be best to avoid high-fat foods and stick to low-fat options like fruits and vegetables.

You can also blend the ingredients in a blender If you don't have a juicer and then strain the mixture using a fine mesh strainer or cheesecloth to remove any pulp.

Blueberry and spinach smoothie.

Ingredients:

1 cup blueberries, fresh or frozen

1 cup spinach leaves, fresh

1 banana

1/2 cup Greek yogurt, plain

1/2 cup almond milk, unsweetened

1/2 teaspoon honey (optional)

Instructions:

Rinse the blueberries and spinach leaves well.

The banana should be peeled.

Combine the blueberries, spinach, banana, Greek yogurt, almond milk, and honey in a blender (if using).

On high speed, blend until smooth and creamy.

Pour into a glass and serve right away.

Please check with your doctor or a dietitian to see if this smoothie is acceptable for your unique needs and dietary limitations connected to pancreatitis.

Carrot, apple, and turmeric juice.

Ingredients:

4 large peeled and sliced carrots

2 cored and diced apples 1/2-inch fresh turmeric root, peeled 1/2 inch peeled fresh ginger root (optional)

1/4 teaspoon black pepper (optional)

Instructions:

If using, peel and cut the carrots, apples, turmeric, and ginger.

Process the carrots, apples, turmeric, ginger, and black pepper (if using) in a juicer until smooth.

If you don't have a juicer, combine the ingredients in a blender and drain the juice through a fine mesh sieve.

Pour the juice into a glass and serve right away.

Consult your doctor or a dietitian to decide if this juice is acceptable for your unique needs and dietary limitations due to pancreatitis. Also, because too much turmeric can cause gastrointestinal distress, it's best to start with a small amount and gradually increase your intake.

Almond milk, banana, and spinach smoothie.

Ingredients:

1 banana

2 cups of fresh spinach leaves

1 cup unsweetened almond milk

1/4 cup plain Greek yogurt

1/2 teaspoon honey (optional)

Instructions:

Peel the banana.

Rinse the spinach leaves.

In a blender, combine the banana, spinach, almond milk, Greek yogurt, and honey (if using).

Blend on high speed until smooth and creamy.

Pour the smoothie into a glass and enjoy it immediately.

Note: Consult your doctor or a dietitian to determine if this smoothie is appropriate for your specific needs and dietary restrictions related to your pancreatitis. Additionally, spinach contains oxalates, which can be harmful for some people with kidney problems, so it's recommended to consume it in moderation.

Cucumber, celery, and mint juice.

Ingredients:

2 cucumbers, peeled and chopped

4 stalks of celery, washed and chopped

1/4 cup fresh mint leaves

1 lemon, juiced

1/4 teaspoon ground black pepper (optional)

Instructions:

Peel and chop the cucumbers and celery.

Rinse the mint leaves.

In a juicer, process the cucumbers, celery, mint leaves, lemon juice, and black pepper (if using) until smooth.

If a juicer is not available, you can blend them in a blender and strain the juice through a fine-mesh sieve.

Pour the juice into a glass and enjoy it immediately.

Note: Be sure to consult with your doctor or a dietitian to determine if this juice is appropriate for your specific needs and dietary restrictions. Celery is known to have a diuretic effect; consuming it in large amounts may lead to an electrolyte imbalance, so it's advisable to consume it in moderation.

Strawberry and kale smoothie.

Ingredients:

1 cup fresh or frozen strawberries

2 cups of fresh kale leaves

1 banana

1/2 cup unsweetened almond milk

1/2 cup plain Greek yogurt

1/2 teaspoon honey (optional)

Instructions:

Rinse the strawberries and kale leaves.

Peel the banana.

In a blender, combine the strawberries, kale, banana, almond milk, Greek yogurt, and honey (if using).

Blend on high speed until smooth and creamy.

Pour the smoothie into a glass and enjoy it immediately.

Note: Consult your doctor or a dietitian to determine if this smoothie is related to your pancreatitis diet. Kale is high in Vitamin K, which can interact with blood-thinning medication, so it's important to check with your doctor if this is something you're taking.

Ginger tea.

Ingredients:

1-inch piece of fresh ginger root, peeled and thinly sliced

2 cups of water

Honey or lemon (optional)

Instructions:

Peel and thinly slice the ginger root.

Bring 2 cups of water to a boil in a small saucepan.

Add the ginger slices to the water and reduce the heat to low.

Let the ginger steep for 10–15 minutes, or until the tea has a strong ginger flavor.

Strain the tea into a mug, discarding the ginger slices.

Add honey or lemon for taste if desired.

Enjoy your tea while it is still warm.

Note: Ginger tea may help to reduce inflammation and pain associated with pancreatitis, but it's important not to consume excessive amounts as it can cause stomach upset.

Peppermint tea.

Ingredients:

1-2 tsp dried peppermint leaves

2 cups of water

Honey or lemon (optional)

Instructions:

Bring 2 cups of water to a boil in a small saucepan.

Add the peppermint leaves to the water and reduce the heat to low.

Let the peppermint steep for 5–7 minutes, or until the tea has a strong peppermint flavor.

Strain the tea into a mug, discarding the leaves.

Add honey or lemon for taste if desired.

Enjoy your tea while it is still warm.

Note: Peppermint tea may help to reduce inflammation and pain associated with pancreatitis, but it's important not to consume excessive amounts as it can cause stomach upset. Peppermint tea can also relax the sphincter between the stomach and esophagus, which can lead to acid reflux symptoms if you already have this condition.

Juices, smoothies, and teas can help with pancreatitis management by delivering critical nutrients and antioxidants while being easy to take. However, you should speak with a doctor or a dietitian to confirm that the components you use are appropriate for your individual needs and dietary It's also worth noting that eating too much of some ingredients, such as ginger or peppermint, might induce gastrointestinal trouble.

Furthermore, drinking large volumes of juice or smoothies might increase sugar intake; therefore, it is advisable to eat in moderation and to include a variety of fruits and vegetables. Drinking beverages such as herbal teas can also be beneficial, although excessive consumption should be avoided.

CHAPTER 10

Tips for Eating Out and Traveling on a Pancreatitis Diet

Eating out and traveling might be difficult for those on a pancreatitis diet. Pancreatitis is a disorder that affects the pancreas, an organ that produces enzymes that aid in food digestion. A pancreatitis diet often consists of avoiding high-fat, high-sugar, and high-protein foods and eating smaller, more frequent meals. Here are some recommendations about dining out and traveling while on a pancreatitis diet:

Pre-research restaurants.

When you research restaurants ahead of time, you are taking the time to seek out eateries before going out to dine. By doing so, you may ensure that you select a restaurant that provides healthy, low-fat selections that are appropriate for your pancreatitis diet. This is significant since consuming high-fat, high-sugar, and high-protein diets can aggravate pancreatitis symptoms and induce more pancreatic inflammation.

When investigating restaurants, look for eateries that serve salads, grilled fish, and steamed veggies. These recipes are often lower in fat and calories, making them an excellent choice for individuals on a pancreatitis diet. You can also look for restaurants that specialize in vegetarian or vegan cuisine, as these meals are typically lower in fat and cholesterol.

It's also a good idea to avoid eateries that serve fried or oily items. Fried meals, such as fried chicken or French fries, are often prepared with a lot of oil, which can be heavy in fat and calories. This can be dangerous for people who have pancreatitis since high-fat meals can aggravate symptoms and make it difficult for the pancreas to digest food adequately. You can lower your chances of experiencing symptoms related to your disease by avoiding these sorts of eateries.

Communicate with your server as follows.

When eating out on a pancreatitis diet, communicating with your server is critical. It is critical to inform your server of any dietary restrictions and particular meal requests so that they may assist you in finding foods that are appropriate for your condition.

It's better to be detailed and clear about what you can and cannot eat when informing your server of your dietary limitations. For instance, you could state something like, "Because I have a pancreatic issue, I must avoid foods that are high in fat, sugar, or protein." "Can you propose some low-fat, easy-to-digest dishes?" By sharing this information with your server, they will be able to offer pancreatitis-friendly foods.

You can also ask your server for advice on dishes that are pancreatitis-friendly. They may be able to recommend low-fat menu options such as grilled fish or steamed veggies. Furthermore, waitresses can inform you about the ingredients and preparation processes of each dish, which might help you pick what to eat.

It's also a good idea to let the kitchen staff know if you have any food allergies so that they can take the necessary precautions to avoid cross-contamination.

You can feel more confident in your meal choices and enjoy your dining experience without jeopardizing your health by interacting with your waitress and asking for recommendations.

Make your food unique.

Customizing your meal is an efficient way to ensure that the food you eat is appropriate for your pancreatitis diet. One method is to request sauces and dressings on the side. In this manner, you may limit the quantity of extra fats and sugar you consume. You can also request a lighter version of the sauce or dressing or ask whether the meal can be prepared without any sauce or dressing.

Another method to personalize your dish is to request that it be prepared with as little oil and butter as possible. Many restaurants cook with a lot of oil and butter, which can raise the fat content of a dish. You can minimize the amount of fat you consume by requesting that your food be prepared with less oil and butter, which is excellent for those with pancreatitis.

You can also request that your food be prepared using a specific method, such as steamed, grilled, or baked. These cooking methods often use less oil and butter and are healthier solutions for people suffering from pancreatitis.

It's important to note that restaurants may not be able to accommodate all requests, but it's worth asking because it's a good way to ensure that the food you're eating is appropriate for your pancreatitis diet and will allow you to enjoy your dinner without jeopardizing your health.

Pack your own snacks.

Packing your own snacks when traveling is a terrific way to guarantee you have healthy options available, even if you can't find them at your destination. This is especially crucial for individuals on a pancreatitis diet, as it can be difficult to obtain low-fat, sugar-free, and protein-rich items when traveling.

Fruits such as apples, berries, and citrus fruits are excellent choices for nutritious snacking. Fruits are high in vitamins, minerals, and antioxidants while being low in fat and calories. Almonds, walnuts, and cashews are other excellent choices. They are high in protein and healthy fats. Furthermore, low-fat crackers are a fantastic source of complex carbs and can be paired with low-fat cheese or hummus for a healthy and enjoyable snack.

When packing your own snacks, ensure that they are easy to transport and do not require refrigeration. To keep perishable snacks fresh, bring along a small cooler or insulated bag.

By bringing your own snacks, you'll have healthy options available even if you can't locate them at your destination. This will allow you to stay on your pancreatitis diet while also enjoying your vacation without jeopardizing your health.

Stay hydrated.

Staying hydrated is essential for overall health, and it is especially critical for people suffering with pancreatitis. The pancreas is important for digestion and enzyme production, and staying hydrated can help support these tasks.

When you are dehydrated, your body has a more difficult time digesting meals and absorbing nutrients, putting additional strain on the pancreas. Staying hydrated allows your body to digest meals more efficiently, reducing the stress on the pancreas.

Water is the best way to stay hydrated because it has no calories, sugar, or caffeine. Aim for 8–10 cups of water each day, with more if you are physically active or in hot weather. Other hydrating fluids to consider are herbal teas, coconut water, and sugar-free electrolyte beverages.

It is also crucial to note that alcohol and caffeine usage should be limited because they can dehydrate you. Sugary drinks should also be avoided because they can aggravate pancreatitis symptoms.

Staying hydrated can assist in promoting pancreatic function, enhancing digestion, and preserving general health. This is especially crucial when eating out or traveling, as it is easy to overlook your hydration needs in unfamiliar surroundings.

You may make eating out and traveling on a pancreatitis diet more comfortable by following these recommendations, and you can enjoy your meals without jeopardizing your health.

CHAPTER 11

Managing Pancreatitis Flare-Ups with Diet.

Pancreatitis is a painful and incapacitating illness that arises when the pancreas gets inflamed. Diet is one of the most efficient strategies to manage pancreatitis flare-ups. You can minimize inflammation, promote the healing process, and avoid future flare-ups by making dietary modifications.

Pancreatitis patients should follow a low-fat, low-sugar, and low-protein diet. Fruits, vegetables, lean meats, and whole grains are examples of such foods. Foods heavy in fat, sugar, and protein, such as fried foods, processed foods, and red meats, should be avoided.

Aside from dietary adjustments, it is also critical to stay hydrated and minimize alcohol and caffeine usage. Drinking enough water can help maintain pancreatic function and enhance digestion.

Working closely with your healthcare physician to build a personalized food plan that is tailored to your individual needs is also essential. They may advise you to take additional nutrients or use drugs to help control your symptoms.

Overall, using food to manage pancreatitis flare-ups can be an effective method to reduce inflammation, aid in healing, and avoid future flare-ups. You may take control of your condition and enhance your general health by making dietary changes, staying hydrated, and limiting certain substances.

Maintaining a low-fat diet.

Pancreatitis flare-ups can result in symptoms such as abdominal pain, nausea, vomiting, and diarrhea. One way to treat these symptoms and prevent future flare-ups is to eat a low-fat diet.

Low-fat pancreatitis diets include avoiding high-fat foods that can strain the pancreas and cause an attack. Fried foods, processed foods, and red meat are examples of diets high in harmful fats that might raise the chance of getting pancreatitis. Individuals suffering from pancreatitis should instead focus on consuming lean meats, whole grains, and enough fruits and vegetables to acquire the nutrients they require without overloading their pancreas.

Finally, a low-fat diet is essential for treating pancreatitis flare-ups. Individuals with pancreatitis can lessen their symptoms, prevent further flare-ups, and enhance their general health and well-being by avoiding high-fat foods and focusing on healthier options.

Restrict your intake of sugary foods and drinks.

Consuming too much sugar can aggravate these symptoms and precipitate a pancreatitis flare-up.

Sugar is a carbohydrate that the body quickly digests, releasing a lot of glucose into the bloodstream. This increase in glucose levels can put additional strain on the pancreas, causing it to work harder and potentially triggering a pancreatitis flare-up. Furthermore, sugar is frequently included in processed and high-fat diets, which can be difficult for the pancreas to handle and contribute to pancreatitis development.

It is critical to limit your intake of sugary meals and drinks to avoid worsening pancreatitis symptoms. Avoiding sugary drinks like soda and fruit juice, as well as sweets like candy and cakes, is part of this. Individuals suffering from pancreatitis should instead focus on eating a well-balanced diet rich in complex carbohydrates, lean proteins, and healthy fats, while limiting their intake of processed and high-fat meals.

Finally, minimizing your sugar intake is a crucial element of controlling pancreatitis symptoms. Individuals with pancreatitis can lower their risk of flare-ups, relieve their symptoms, and maintain better overall health by avoiding sugary foods and drinks.

Reduce protein intake.

The pancreas aids digestion by creating digestive enzymes that help break down food into smaller components that can be absorbed by the body. When high-protein foods are ingested in large quantities, the pancreas must manufacture more digestive enzymes to breakdown them, putting more load on the organ and perhaps causing harm. High-protein diets may also cause the development of illnesses such as pancreatitis, which is inflammation of the pancreas, in some people.

Individuals with specific medical disorders, such as pancreatitis or pancreatic insufficiency, should limit their protein consumption for these reasons in order to lessen the burden on the pancreas and prevent additional damage to the organ. This may entail restricting their intake of high-protein foods and replacing them with lean protein sources that are simpler for the pancreas to digest, such as fish and poultry.

While lowering protein intake may be advantageous for people with certain medical issues, it is still a vital component that the body needs for development, repair, and overall health. A doctor or trained dietitian should be consulted to establish the right amount of protein for each individual based on their specific needs and health status.

Increase your intake of fruits and vegetables.

Consuming more fruits and vegetables is beneficial to one's general health and well-being. They are high in important vitamins, minerals, and fiber while being low in calories. Here are some reasons why you should increase your intake:

Fruits and vegetables are high in vital vitamins and minerals such as vitamin C, A, and K, as well as folate, potassium, and iron.

Fruits and vegetables are low in calories and high in fiber, which makes them filling and aids in weight management.

Improves Digestion: The fiber in fruits and vegetables encourages regular bowel movements, which reduces the risk of constipation and other digestive issues.

Reduces the Risk of Chronic Diseases: Eating more fruits and vegetables has been linked to a lower risk of chronic diseases like heart disease, stroke, and several types of cancer.

Boosts Immune System: Fruits and vegetables are high in antioxidants and nutrients that aid in the proper functioning of the immune system.

To improve your intake of fruits and vegetables, try them as snacks, include them in meals, and make them a staple of your diet. Attempt to consume at least 5 servings of fruits and vegetables per day.

Consume whole grains.

During flare-ups, it's critical to eat meals that are easy on the digestive system and don't place extra strain on the pancreas.

People with pancreatitis should eat whole grains, including quinoa, brown rice, and oats. Complex carbohydrates, which differ from simple carbohydrates in that they are made up of longer chains of sugar molecules, are abundant in these grains. As a result, complex carbs digest more slowly and give a slow, consistent supply of energy rather than a rapid surge followed by a crash.

Whole grains are a good source of fiber in addition to delivering sustained energy. Fiber is beneficial to digestive health because it helps regulate bowel movements, lowering the risk of constipation and other digestive problems.

While whole grains can be beneficial for people with pancreatitis, they should be consumed in moderation. Eating a lot of carbs of any kind might place a load on the pancreas and potentially increase symptoms.

Finally, introducing nutritious grains like quinoa, brown rice, and oats into the diet during pancreatitis flare-ups can provide long-lasting energy and improve digestive health. However, it is critical to take these items in moderation and adhere to any dietary instructions prescribed by a healthcare expert.

Drink plenty of water.

Drinking enough water is essential for maintaining proper pancreatic function and digestion, especially during pancreatitis flare-ups. The pancreas is a gland that is essential for digestion and blood sugar management. When the pancreas is inflamed, it might be difficult for it to operate regularly, resulting in digestion issues and other symptoms.

Drinking plenty of water to stay hydrated can help the pancreas work more effectively. Water is necessary for digestion because it aids in the breakdown of food and its passage through the digestive tract. Dehydration causes digestion to become sluggish and inefficient, putting additional load on the pancreas.

Furthermore, drinking water can aid in the removal of toxins and waste products from the body, lowering the risk of infection and other issues. This is especially critical during pancreatitis flare-ups since an inflamed pancreas may not be able to remove waste as efficiently as it typically would.

It is crucial to note that drinking too much water can be harmful because it dilutes the body's electrolytes and disrupts fluid balance. This can aggravate pancreatitis symptoms and potentially lead to complications.

To summarize, drinking sufficient amounts of water is essential for maintaining normal pancreatic function and assisting digestion during pancreatitis flare-ups. However, it is critical to drink enough water to be hydrated but not so much that it upsets the body's fluid equilibrium. Consult a healthcare provider for personalized fluid intake recommendations.

Limit your intake of alcohol and caffeine.

It is critical to minimize alcohol and caffeine consumption during pancreatitis flare-ups. These drugs can have a detrimental impact on the pancreas and aggravate symptoms.

Alcohol is a common cause of pancreatitis because it irritates and inflames the pancreas. Furthermore, alcohol is a diuretic, which means it increases the quantity of fluid lost from the body through urine.

This can cause dehydration, which can increase pancreatitis symptoms and make it more difficult for the pancreas to function correctly.

Caffeine is another substance that might be harmful to people who have pancreatitis. Caffeine is a stimulant that can raise blood pressure and pulse rate, putting additional strain on the pancreas. Caffeine, like alcohol, is a diuretic and can cause dehydration. Dehydration can exacerbate pancreatitis symptoms and potentially lead to complications.

During pancreatitis flare-ups, it is critical to limit your intake of alcohol and caffeine. This may imply eliminating these substances completely or restricting their use to a limited amount. Consult a healthcare provider for individualized advice on alcohol and caffeine consumption.

Finally, restricting alcohol and caffeine consumption is critical for treating pancreatitis symptoms during flare-ups. These drugs can dehydrate the body and irritate the pancreas, making regular function more difficult. Consult a healthcare provider for individualized advice on alcohol and caffeine consumption.

Collaboration with a healthcare professional.

Collaboration with a healthcare practitioner is essential for controlling pancreatitis symptoms during flare-ups. Your healthcare practitioner can assist you in developing a personalized nutrition plan that is suited to your specific needs, taking into account things like your current health state, medications, and lifestyle.

A personalized nutrition plan can assist you in managing pancreatitis symptoms by ensuring that you are obtaining the nutrients you require to maintain good health and reduce the risk of complications. This could include advice on which foods to eat or avoid, as well as guidance on portion sizes and meal times.

In addition, your doctor may urge you to consume more nutrients or use medications to help reduce your symptoms. For example, they may advise taking digestive health supplements such as probiotics or digestive enzymes. They may also prescribe drugs to help control pancreatitis-related pain, inflammation, or other problems.

Working collaboratively with your healthcare provider to develop a personalized nutrition plan that suits your specific needs is critical. This can help ensure that you are managing your symptoms and reducing the risk of problems.

Collaborating with a healthcare expert is a key element of controlling pancreatitis symptoms during flare-ups. A customized dietary plan, in conjunction with supplementary nutrients or drugs, can help you regulate your symptoms and maintain your health. Consult a healthcare provider for personalized treatment advice and options.

CHAPTER 12

Supplements and Herbs for Pancreatitis.

Individuals suffering from pancreatitis can benefit from the use of supplements and herbs as complementary therapies. These complementary therapies can aid with the body's natural healing processes, as well as lessen symptoms and enhance general health. However, not all vitamins and herbs are healthy for people with pancreatitis, and some may mix with drugs or other treatments. Before beginning any new vitamins or herbs, it is critical to consult with a healthcare practitioner, especially if you have any underlying health concerns or are using any prescription drugs.

Collaboration with a healthcare practitioner is essential for controlling pancreatitis symptoms during flare-ups. Your healthcare practitioner can assist you in developing a personalized nutrition plan that is suited to your specific needs, taking into account things like your current health state, medications, and lifestyle.

A personalized nutrition plan can assist you in managing pancreatitis symptoms by ensuring that you are obtaining the nutrients you require to maintain good health and reduce the risk of complications. This could include advice on which foods to eat or avoid, as well as guidance on portion sizes and meal times.

Your doctor may urge you to consume more nutrients or use medications to help reduce your symptoms. For example, they may advise taking digestive health supplements such as probiotics or digestive enzymes. They may also prescribe drugs to help control pancreatitis-related pain, inflammation, or other problems.

Working collaboratively with your healthcare provider to develop a personalized nutrition plan that suits your specific needs is critical. This can help ensure that you are managing your symptoms and reducing the risk of problems.

A customized dietary plan, in conjunction with supplementary nutrients or drugs, can help you regulate your symptoms and maintain your health. Consult a healthcare provider for personalized treatment advice and options.

Probiotics.

Probiotics are live microorganisms like bacteria and yeast that are taken as a supplement. They are believed to benefit digestive health by promoting the balance of beneficial gut flora. Pancreatitis can alter the gut flora, or the microorganisms that live in the digestive tract, resulting in digestive symptoms such as bloating, gas, and constipation.

When the gut flora is out of balance, it increases the risk of additional health issues like infections, inflammation, and digestive disorders. Probiotics can help restore gut flora balance and enhance digestive health, reducing symptoms and improving general well-being in people with pancreatitis.

Probiotics can also help support the body's natural defense mechanisms by creating antibacterial compounds. They can also help strengthen the immune system, which can guard against infections and other health issues.

Finally, probiotics can help with digestive health and enhance gut flora, which can be disrupted in people with pancreatitis. They can aid in the reduction of symptoms, the improvement of overall well-being, and the support of the body's natural defense mechanisms. Before taking any probiotics, consult with a healthcare expert to ensure that they are safe and appropriate for you.

Digestive enzymes.

Digestive enzymes are naturally occurring molecules in the body that aid in the digestion of food by breaking it down into smaller, more readily digested bits. Pancreatitis causes the pancreas to generate insufficient digestive enzymes, resulting in symptoms such as bloating, gas, and constipation.

Digestive enzymes can help boost the digestive process and alleviate discomfort. Digestive enzyme supplements often contain a blend of enzymes that aid in the breakdown of various types of food, such as carbs, proteins, and lipids.

By enhancing the digestion process, digestive enzyme supplements can help alleviate symptoms such as bloating, gas, and constipation. This can also help lower the pancreas' workload, allowing it to recover and minimize inflammation.

Finally, digestive enzymes can support the digestive process and alleviate symptoms like bloating, gas, and constipation in people with pancreatitis. They can help enhance digestion and lessen the pancreas' burden, allowing it to recover and minimize inflammation. Before taking digestive enzyme supplements, contact a healthcare expert because they may interfere with other medications or medical problems.

Omega-3 fatty acids.

Omega-3 fatty acids are a form of polyunsaturated fat with anti-inflammatory effects. They can be found in fish such as salmon and mackerel, as well as in plant-based sources such as flaxseeds and chia seeds.

Inflammation can be a major contributor to symptoms and overall health in people with pancreatitis. Omega-3 fatty acids, by lowering inflammation, can improve general health and alleviate symptoms in people with pancreatitis.

John, a 50-year-old male, had been suffering from pancreatitis for some years. He experienced regular flare-ups that caused abdominal pain, nausea, and vomiting. After consulting with his doctor, John decided to increase his intake of omega-3 fatty acids by eating more fish and taking a daily omega-3 supplement. After a few weeks, John's symptoms and overall health had significantly improved.

Kimberly, a 35-year-old woman, was diagnosed with pancreatitis after experiencing acute abdominal pain. Her doctor advised her to take an omega-3 supplement to minimize inflammation and improve her general health. She observed that her symptoms had improved and she was having fewer flare-ups after several months of using the supplement.

Finally, omega-3 fatty acids have been shown to lower inflammation and enhance general health in people with pancreatitis. They can also provide a variety of other health benefits and may help lessen the risk of developing other health issues. Before taking omega-3 supplements, contact a healthcare expert because they may interfere with other medications or medical problems.

Vitamin B12.

Vitamin B12 is a necessary component that aids in the functioning of the pancreas and the maintenance of energy levels. The pancreas is an important organ that generates digestive enzymes and hormones that regulate blood sugar levels, such as insulin.

Vitamin B12 levels in pancreatitis patients may be low due to decreased production of intrinsic factor, a chemical produced in the stomach that is essential for vitamin B12 absorption. Anemia, fatigue, and issues with the nervous system can all result from a shortage of vitamin B12.

For example, Bob, a 45-year-old man suffering from pancreatitis, was frequently fatigued and exhausted. He was diagnosed with vitamin B12 insufficiency after speaking with his doctor. He was recommended a daily vitamin B12 supplement and began eating more vitamin B12-rich foods such as meat, chicken, fish, and dairy items. Bob observed a considerable improvement in his energy levels and overall well-being after a few months.

Jane, a 55-year-old lady with pancreatitis who was experiencing weariness and weakness, is another case in point. She was identified as having a vitamin

B12 deficiency after a blood test. Her doctor advised her to take a daily vitamin B12 pill and eat more vitamin B12-rich foods. Jane took her doctor's advice and saw a substantial improvement in her energy levels and overall well-being after a few months.

Finally, vitamin B12 can assist in promoting pancreatic function and increasing energy levels in people with pancreatitis. A shortage of vitamin B12 can cause anemia, exhaustion, and nervous system disorders, so include vitamin B12-rich foods in your diet and consult with a healthcare practitioner about taking a daily supplement if necessary.

Glutamine.

Glutamine is an amino acid that is essential for gut lining health and inflammation control. The gut lining can become damaged in people with pancreatitis, causing inflammation and increased permeability, which can lead to nutrient deficiencies, digestive difficulties, and systemic inflammation.

Mark, a 35-year-old man with pancreatitis, was suffering from acute abdominal discomfort and digestive difficulties. He was recommended a daily glutamine supplement after speaking with his doctor. Mark also altered his diet, limiting his intake of processed foods and increasing his intake of anti-inflammatory items. Mark saw a considerable improvement in his digestive issues and overall well-being after many months of taking the supplement and making dietary changes.

Sarah, a 40-year-old woman with pancreatitis who was experiencing abdominal pain, bloating, and constipation, is another case in point. She was provided a daily glutamine supplement and made dietary changes to minimize her intake of inflammatory foods and increase her consumption of anti-inflammatory foods after speaking with her doctor. Sarah saw a dramatic improvement in her digestive issues and overall well-being after many months of taking the supplement and making dietary changes.

Finally, glutamine can help promote the health of the gut lining and reduce inflammation in people who have pancreatitis. Incorporating glutamine-rich foods such as grass-fed beef, chicken, fish, and dairy products into your diet, as well as speaking with a healthcare expert about taking a daily glutamine supplement, can help improve digestive symptoms and general well-being.

Milk Thistle.

Milk thistle is an herb that has been used for millennia to help with liver function and overall health. The liver and pancreas operate closely together in people with pancreatitis, so any abnormalities with the pancreas can affect the liver. Milk thistle is thought to contain antioxidant qualities, which may help protect and improve liver function.

David, a 50-year-old man with pancreatitis, for example, was having liver difficulties as a result of his disease. He was prescribed a daily Milk Thistle supplement after speaking with his doctor. In addition to taking the pill, David altered his diet, cutting back on processed foods and boosting his intake of anti-inflammatory items. David saw a considerable increase in his liver function and overall well-being after several months of taking the supplement and making dietary modifications.

Emily, a 45-year-old woman with pancreatitis, was also dealing with liver issues as a result of her condition. She was provided a daily Milk Thistle supplement and made dietary changes to minimize her intake of inflammatory foods and increase her consumption of anti-inflammatory foods after speaking with her doctor. Emily saw a dramatic increase in her liver function and overall well-being after several months of taking the supplement and making dietary changes.

Finally, milk thistle contains antioxidant qualities and may enhance liver function in those with pancreatitis. Incorporating Milk Thistle-rich foods like dandelion greens and artichokes into your diet, as well as consulting with a healthcare expert about taking a daily Milk Thistle supplement, can enhance liver function and your general well-being.

Curcumin.

Curcumin, a chemical found in the spice turmeric, has anti-inflammatory properties. Inflammation is a typical problem in people with pancreatitis, and it can cause a variety of symptoms such as abdominal discomfort, bloating, and diarrhea. Adding turmeric to your diet or taking a curcumin supplement can help reduce inflammation and enhance overall health.

Jack, a 40-year-old man with pancreatitis who was suffering from a variety of symptoms such as inflammation and abdominal pain. Jack was instructed by his doctor to take a daily curcumin tablet and to add turmeric to his diet. Jack began using turmeric in his cooking and began taking a curcumin supplement on a daily basis. After a few weeks, Jack observed a considerable improvement in his symptoms, including less inflammation and stomach pain.

Finally, curcumin, a chemical found in turmeric, has anti-inflammatory qualities that can help reduce inflammation and improve overall health in people suffering from pancreatitis. Under the supervision of a healthcare expert, incorporating turmeric into your diet and taking a curcumin supplement can help to lessen symptoms and enhance overall well-being.

Ginger.

Ginger is a root vegetable that is widely used in both cooking and medicine. It has been used in traditional medicine for thousands of years to cure a variety of diseases such as nausea, digestive difficulties, and inflammation.

Nausea: Ginger is frequently used to treat nausea, particularly morning sickness during pregnancy. It works by preventing the brain from sending impulses that cause nausea. A study found that consuming ginger before chemotherapy can help cancer patients reduce nausea. One woman claimed that drinking ginger tea helped her overcome pregnancy sickness.

Ginger has been demonstrated to promote digestive function and boost nutritional absorption. It's also used to treat bloating, gas, and other digestive issues. A man claimed that eating ginger before meals helped his digestion and reduced bloating.

It contains anti-inflammatory effects and has been used to treat pain and swelling caused by disorders such as osteoarthritis. It works by preventing the body from producing specific inflammatory chemicals. A rheumatoid arthritis patient claimed that using ginger supplements reduced joint discomfort and edema.

To summarize, ginger provides a variety of health benefits, including the ability to alleviate nausea, enhance digestion, and reduce inflammation. It is available fresh, powdered, as an oil or juice, and as a supplement. However, before using ginger as a remedy for any medical issue, please consult with a healthcare expert.

Slippery Elm.

The bark of the Slippery Elm tree, which is native to North America, is used to manufacture therapeutic beverages and supplements. For generations, it has been used to relax the digestive tract and treat digestive issues such as bloating, gas, and constipation.

Pancreatitis is characterized by pancreatic inflammation, which can result in digestive symptoms such as bloating, gas, and constipation. By coating and calming the digestive tract, Slippery Elm can help alleviate gastrointestinal symptoms. The mucilage in Slippery Elm functions as a natural lubricant, allowing food and waste to flow more easily through the digestive system.

According to one study, Slippery Elm can help relieve symptoms of irritable bowel syndrome

(IBS), which is characterized by bloating, gas, and constipation. One individual stated that drinking Slippery Elm tea helped her with IBS-related bloating and gas. Another pancreatitis patient said that using Slippery Elm tablets helped him with constipation and bloating.

Finally, Slippery Elm can help relax the digestive tract and alleviate symptoms of pancreatitis such as bloating, gas, and constipation. It can be drunk as tea, taken as a supplement, or mixed with meals. However, before using Slippery Elm, contact your healthcare provider, especially if you are taking other medications, as it may interfere with their absorption.

Licorice Root.

Licorice Root is a plant native to Europe and Asia that has been used in traditional medicine for thousands of years for a variety of purposes, including lowering inflammation, supporting digestive health, and promoting general well-being.

Pancreatitis is an inflammation of the pancreas that can cause digestive issues and discomfort. By inhibiting the formation of some inflammatory substances, licorice root can help reduce inflammation in the body, including the pancreas. It has also been demonstrated to benefit digestive health by increasing the production of digestive fluids and enzymes, thereby alleviating digestive symptoms such as bloating, gas, and constipation.

Licorice root also has a relaxing impact on the digestive tract, which aids in the relief of stomach discomfort symptoms. It has also been used to stimulate the immune system and reduce stress, thus improving general well-being.

According to one study, licorice root can help lessen the symptoms of peptic ulcers, which are commonly caused by digestive tract inflammation. One man said that consuming licorice root pills helped him improve pancreatitis symptoms such as bloating, gas, and constipation. Another woman with IBS found that drinking licorice root tea relieved her bloating and gas problems.

Finally, in pancreatitis, licorice root can help reduce inflammation, enhance digestive health, and improve overall well-being. It can be drunk as tea, taken as a supplement, or mixed with meals. However, before using licorice root, contact a healthcare provider because it may interact with some drugs and have negative effects in excessive dosages.

It should be noted that these supplements and herbs should only be used under the supervision of a healthcare practitioner. Some supplements are not suitable for everyone, while others may interfere with prescriptions or other therapies. Before beginning any new supplements or herbs, consult with a healthcare practitioner, especially if you have any underlying health concerns or are using any prescription drugs.

CHAPTER 13

Frequently Asked Questions about the Pancreatitis Diet.

Pancreatitis is an inflammation of the pancreas, an organ important for digestion, enzyme synthesis, and insulin regulation. Pancreatitis symptoms include abdominal pain, nausea, vomiting, and digestive issues. A healthy diet is critical for treating these symptoms and aiding recovery.

What to eat, what to avoid, and how to maintain enough nutrient intake are frequently asked questions about the pancreatitis diet. Some often asked questions include: "Can I eat fatty foods?" What are the best protein sources? How can I ensure that I obtain adequate vitamins and minerals? These questions highlight the importance of a well-balanced, nutrient-dense diet for people suffering from pancreatitis. Understanding the specific dietary needs and limits associated with this illness might assist individuals in making informed food choices.

What is pancreatitis?

Pancreatitis is a condition in which the pancreas, an organ involved in digestion and insulin regulation, becomes inflamed.

What are the symptoms of pancreatitis?

Symptoms of pancreatitis can include abdominal pain, nausea, vomiting, and digestive problems.

Why is diet important for those with pancreatitis?

A proper diet is essential for managing the symptoms of pancreatitis and promoting recovery.

Can I eat fatty foods with pancreatitis?

It is recommended to limit the intake of fatty foods, as they can worsen symptoms of pancreatitis.

What are the best sources of protein for those with pancreatitis?

Lean protein sources, such as chicken, fish, and tofu, are recommended for those with pancreatitis.

Is it okay to eat spicy foods with pancreatitis?

Spicy foods can irritate the digestive system and worsen symptoms of pancreatitis, so it is recommended to avoid or limit them.

Can I drink alcohol with pancreatitis?

Alcohol should be avoided as it can worsen symptoms and slow down the healing process.

What should I eat for breakfast with pancreatitis?

A balanced breakfast with whole grain carbohydrates, lean protein, and healthy fats can provide the nutrients and energy needed to start the day.

Can I eat dairy products with pancreatitis?

Some people with pancreatitis may be able to tolerate dairy products in small amounts, while others may need to avoid them completely.

How can I make sure I am getting enough vitamins and minerals with pancreatitis?

Eating a varied diet with plenty of fruits and vegetables, lean protein, and whole grains can help ensure adequate nutrient intake.

What are the best foods for relieving digestive symptoms in pancreatitis?

Foods that are easy to digest and low in fat, such as boiled potatoes, rice, and soup, can help relieve digestive symptoms in pancreatitis.

Can I eat high-fiber foods with pancreatitis?

High-fiber foods can be difficult to digest for some people with pancreatitis and may worsen symptoms, so it is recommended to limit or avoid them.

What are the best liquids to drink with pancreatitis?

Clear liquids, such as water, broth, and herbal tea, can help keep the body hydrated and relieve digestive symptoms.

Can I eat nuts with pancreatitis?

Nuts are high in fat and may worsen symptoms of pancreatitis, so it is recommended to limit or avoid them.

What are the best snacks for those with pancreatitis?

Snacks that are low in fat and easy to digest, such as apples, carrots, and crackers, can be good choices for those with pancreatitis.

How can I make sure I am getting enough calories with pancreatitis?

Eating small, frequent meals throughout the day can help ensure adequate calorie intake for those with pancreatitis.

What should I eat for dinner with pancreatitis?

A balanced dinner with lean protein, whole grain carbohydrates, and vegetables can provide the nutrients and energy needed for the evening.

Can I eat fried foods with pancreatitis?

Fried foods are high in fat and can worsen symptoms of pancreatitis, so it is recommended to limit or avoid them.

What are the best foods for managing symptoms of abdominal pain in pancreatitis?

Foods that are easy to digest and low in fat, such as boiled potatoes and rice, can help relieve abdominal pain in pancreatitis.

CHAPTER 14

Resources for Further Information and Support

Pancreatitis can be a difficult condition to treat, but there are numerous tools available to assist. There is a plethora of information and support available for people living with pancreatitis, ranging from books and websites to support groups and healthcare specialists. These resources can be helpful if you are looking for information on managing symptoms, establishing a treatment plan, or connecting with others who understand what you are going through. It is possible to successfully treat pancreatitis and live a healthy and fulfilling life with the correct information and assistance.

American Pancreatic Association.

The American Pancreatic Association (APA) is a non-profit organization dedicated to the advancement of pancreatic disease knowledge and awareness. The American Pancreas Association (APA) provides information and services to healthcare professionals, patients, and families affected by pancreatitis and other pancreatic diseases. Through research, teaching, and advocacy, they aim to improve patient outcomes. The APA assists researchers, hosts events and workshops, and aims to promote public knowledge about pancreatic illnesses. They also provide a variety of tools and support services, such as a pancreatic expert referral network, instructional materials, and access to the most recent research and treatment trials. The APA is a valuable resource for anyone seeking information and assistance with pancreatitis management.

Pancreatic Cancer Action Network.

The Pancreatic Cancer Action Network (PanCAN) is a non-profit organization focused on advancing research, patient support, and advocacy for pancreatic cancer. Their mission is to improve patient outcomes and increase survival rates through early detection and effective treatments. PanCAN provides support and resources for patients, families, and healthcare professionals, including a comprehensive website, patient services, and a national support line. They also support pancreatic cancer research through funding and collaborations with leading research institutions. In addition, PanCAN advocates for policies and legislation to increase funding for pancreatic cancer research and improve patient access to quality care. With a strong commitment to patient advocacy, education, and research, PanCAN is a valuable resource for those impacted by pancreatic cancer.

National Pancreas Foundation.

The National Pancreas Foundation (NPF) is a non-profit organization dedicated to improving the lives of people affected by pancreatic illnesses. The NPF provides a range of tools and support services to patients, families, and healthcare professionals, including information and educational materials, a nationwide support network, and a helpline. Additionally, the NPF funds research into pancreatic illnesses and gives support and services for patients, including financial aid, support groups, and access to clinical trials. The NPF is committed to raising awareness of pancreatic disorders, improving patient outcomes, and enhancing information and understanding of these conditions. With a focus on patient advocacy and education, the NPF is a crucial resource for people impacted by pancreatic illnesses.

Mayo Clinic.

The Mayo Clinic is a leading healthcare institution and one of the largest integrated, not-for-profit medical groups in the world. With a focus on patient care, teaching, and research, the Mayo Clinic is a premier resource for anyone seeking information and assistance regarding pancreatitis management. The clinic offers a range of services and resources for patients with pancreatitis, including a team of doctors with expertise in digestive illnesses, a comprehensive library of patient education materials, and access to the newest treatments and research. Patients at the Mayo Clinic can receive a full examination and treatment plan, including food recommendations, medication management, and supportive care services. With a focus on patient-centered treatment and cutting-edge research, the Mayo Clinic is a helpful resource for anyone seeking information and support for pancreatitis management.

WebMD.

WebMD is a renowned health information website that provides information and resources on a wide range of medical ailments, including pancreatitis. The site offers a comprehensive and user-friendly platform for people to learn about their health, including complete information on symptoms, diagnosis, treatment, and management of pancreatitis. WebMD also includes tools and information for tracking and managing one's health, like symptom checks, medication recommendations, and health calculators. In addition to its instructional materials, WebMD offers a community platform where individuals can connect with others, ask questions, and share stories relating to pancreatitis and other health concerns. With a focus on patient education and participation, WebMD is a helpful resource for people seeking information and assistance for pancreatitis care.

American Gastroenterological Association.

The American Gastroenterological Association (AGA) is a professional association representing over 16,000 gastroenterologists and other healthcare professionals in the field of digestive illnesses. The AGA's objective is to promote patient care via research, education, and advocacy. With an emphasis on digestive health, the AGA offers a range of resources and services for healthcare professionals, including educational programs, research funding, and clinical practice guidelines. The AGA also provides information and services for patients, including a comprehensive website and patient education tools. The AGA is a helpful resource for anyone seeking information and assistance for pancreatitis management, as well as for other digestive diseases. With an emphasis on developing the profession of gastroenterology and improving patient outcomes, the AGA is a valuable resource for anyone seeking information and support for pancreatitis and other digestive problems.

National Institute of Diabetes and Digestive and Kidney Diseases.

The National Institute of Diabetes and Digestive and Kidney Diseases (NIDDK) is one of the institutes of the National Institutes of Health (NIH). The NIDDK is dedicated to investigating and improving health and disease management for gut, diabetic, and kidney disorders. With an emphasis on pancreatitis, the NIDDK conducts and funds research into the causes, diagnosis, and treatment of pancreatitis with the objective of improving patient outcomes. The NIDDK also provides information and tools for patients, including a comprehensive website and educational materials. In addition to its research work, the NIDDK is involved in establishing and supporting public health initiatives, such as community-based preventative programs and health awareness campaigns. With an emphasis on promoting science and improving patient outcomes, the NIDDK is a helpful resource for people seeking information and support for pancreatitis care.

Pancreatitis Support Group.

A pancreatitis support group is a community of people brought together by their common experience with pancreatitis. These communities provide a venue for patients to interact, share their experiences, and offer support to one another. Members of a pancreatitis support group may include patients, family members, and friends who are afflicted by the ailment. These meetings give a feeling of community and offer an opportunity for individuals to connect with others who understand the hardships of living with pancreatitis. They also give a platform for exchanging information and discussing treatments, symptoms, and other aspects of the condition. Many pancreatitis support groups are organized by organizations dedicated to improving the lives of pancreatitis patients, such as the National Pancreas Foundation and the American Pancreatic Association. These groups are a wonderful resource for anyone seeking information and support for pancreatitis management and can be a source of comfort and encouragement for those affected by this problem.

American College of Gastroenterology.

The American College of Gastroenterology (ACG) is a professional organization dedicated to developing the science of gastroenterology and improving patient care. The ACG represents nearly 14,000 gastroenterologists and other healthcare professionals in the field of digestive illnesses. With an emphasis on digestive health, the ACG offers a range of resources and services for healthcare professionals, including educational programs, research funding, and clinical practice guidelines. The ACG also provides information and services for patients, including a comprehensive website and patient education tools. The ACG is a helpful resource for anyone seeking information and assistance for pancreatitis management, as well as for other digestive diseases. With an emphasis on developing the profession of gastroenterology and improving patient outcomes, the ACG is a valuable resource for anyone seeking information and assistance for pancreatitis and other digestive problems.

International Association of Pancreatology.

The International Association of Pancreatology (IAP) is a professional association dedicated to developing the subject of pancreatology and enhancing patient treatment. The IAP represents academics, doctors, and healthcare professionals from around the world who are dedicated to expanding knowledge and improving patient outcomes for individuals with pancreatic disorders. The IAP provides a venue for sharing information and developing the subject through research and education efforts. The IAP also provides services for individuals and families impacted by pancreatic diseases, including information on pancreatitis management and access to a network of professionals in the field. With an emphasis on increasing science and improving patient outcomes, the IAP is a vital resource for people seeking information and assistance for pancreatitis care and other pancreatic disorders.

National Institute for Health and Care Excellence.

The National Institute for Health and Care Excellence (NICE) is a national agency in the United Kingdom responsible for giving guidance and advice on the promotion of good health and the prevention and treatment of ill health. NICE develops clinical recommendations, quality standards, and technology appraisals to enable healthcare professionals, consumers, and the public to make educated decisions regarding care and treatment. With a focus on evidence-based practice, NICE provides guidance and recommendations for the management of pancreatitis and other health disorders. NICE also provides information and resources for patients and families affected by pancreatitis and other health disorders, including information on therapies and symptom management. With a focus on promoting good health and improving patient outcomes, NICE is a helpful resource for anyone seeking information and support for pancreatitis management and other health disorders in the United Kingdom.

American Society for Gastrointestinal Endoscopy.

The American Society for Gastrointestinal Endoscopy (ASGE) is a professional organization dedicated to developing the science of gastrointestinal endoscopy and enhancing patient care. The ASGE represents nearly 15,000 healthcare professionals, including gastroenterologists, surgeons, and other specialists in the field of digestive illnesses. With an emphasis on endoscopic treatments, the ASGE offers a range of resources and services for healthcare professionals, including educational programs, research funding, and clinical practice standards. The ASGE also provides information and tools for patients, including a comprehensive website and patient education materials. The ASGE is a great resource for anyone seeking information and support for pancreatitis management, as well as for other digestive disorders, as endoscopy is a common diagnostic and therapeutic tool utilized in the management of pancreatitis. With an emphasis on promoting the area of gastrointestinal endoscopy and improving patient outcomes, the ASGE is a valuable resource for anyone seeking information and assistance for pancreatitis and other digestive illnesses.

Digestive Disease National Coalition.

The Digestive Disease National Coalition (DDNC) is a non-profit organization in the United States dedicated to improving public policy and undertaking advocacy projects pertaining to digestive illnesses. The DDNC represents over 100 patient advocacy and professional groups, including the American College of Gastroenterology and the National Pancreas Foundation. The DDNC fights for policies that promote digestive health, enhance access to care, and boost funding for digestive disease research. The DDNC also provides information and support for individuals and families affected by digestive illnesses, including pancreatitis. With an emphasis on influencing public policy and advocacy for digestive health, the DDNC is a helpful resource for anyone seeking information and assistance for pancreatitis care and other digestive illnesses.

Gastroenterology and Hepatology Journal.

Gastroenterology and Hepatology Publication (GHJ) is a peer-reviewed medical journal that focuses on the latest research and advancements in the domains of gastroenterology and hepatology. The GHJ publishes original research articles, reviews, case reports, and editorials addressing a wide range of topics relevant to digestive health, including pancreatitis. The publication is geared towards healthcare professionals, researchers, and specialists in the fields of gastroenterology and hepatology. The GHJ is a helpful resource for anyone seeking information and support for pancreatitis management, since it gives up-to-date information on the latest research, treatments, and breakthroughs in the field. With an emphasis on promoting knowledge and improving patient outcomes, the Gastroenterology and Hepatology Journal is a significant resource for anyone seeking information and support for pancreatitis and other digestive disorders.

Journal of Pancreatology.

The Journal of Pancreatology is a peer-reviewed medical journal dedicated to the study of pancreatology. The journal offers original research articles, reviews, and case reports covering a wide range of issues relevant to pancreatic disease, including pancreatitis. The Journal of Pancreatology is geared towards healthcare practitioners, researchers, and specialists in the subject of pancreatology. The journal provides up-to-date information on the latest research, treatments, and discoveries in the field of pancreatology, making it a helpful resource for anyone seeking information and support for pancreatitis care. With an emphasis on increasing science and improving patient outcomes, the Journal of Pancreatology is a vital resource for anyone seeking information and support for pancreatitis and other pancreatic problems.

Pancreas Journal.

The Pancreas Publication is a peer-reviewed medical journal dedicated to the study of the pancreas and pancreatic disorders. The journal provides original research articles, reviews, and case reports covering a wide range of topics relating to the pancreas, including pancreatitis. The Pancreas Journal is geared towards healthcare professionals, researchers, and specialists in the subject of pancreatology. The journal provides up-to-date information on the latest research, treatments, and discoveries in the field of pancreatology, making it a helpful resource for anyone seeking information and support for pancreatitis care. With an emphasis on increasing knowledge and improving patient outcomes, the Pancreas Journal is a significant resource for anyone seeking information and support for pancreatitis and other pancreatic disorders.

Pancreatology.

Pancreatology is a peer-reviewed medical journal dedicated to the study of the pancreas and pancreatic disorders. The journal provides original research articles, reviews, and case reports covering a wide range of topics relating to the pancreas, including pancreatitis. Pancreatology is intended for healthcare professionals, researchers, and specialists in the field of pancreatology. The journal provides up-to-date information on the latest research, treatments, and discoveries in the field of pancreatology, making it a helpful resource for anyone seeking information and support for pancreatitis care. With an emphasis on expanding science and improving patient outcomes, pancreatology is a significant resource for anyone seeking information and assistance for pancreatitis and other pancreatic diseases.

Expert Consult Textbook of Pancreatic Surgery.

Expert Consult Textbook of Pancreatic Surgery is a comprehensive medical textbook that covers all elements of pancreatic surgery. The textbook contains in-depth information on the diagnosis, treatment, and management of pancreatic disorders, including pancreatitis. The textbook is directed at healthcare professionals, including surgeons, gastroenterologists, and specialists in the field of pancreatic surgery. The textbook contains thorough information on surgical procedures, postoperative care, and patient outcomes, making it a helpful resource for individuals seeking information and assistance for pancreatitis management. The Expert Consult Textbook of Pancreatic Surgery is a comprehensive and authoritative resource that gives up-to-date information and recommendations on the management of pancreatic illnesses.

The Pancreas: Biology, Pathobiology, and Diseases.

The Pancreas: Biology, Pathobiology, and Pathologies is a comprehensive medical textbook that covers all areas of pancreatic biology and diseases. The textbook contains in-depth information on the anatomy, physiology, and pathophysiology of the pancreas, including pancreatitis. The textbook is intended for healthcare practitioners, researchers, and specialists in the subject of pancreatology. The textbook contains thorough information on the causes, symptoms, diagnosis, and treatment of pancreatic illnesses, making it a helpful resource for anyone seeking information and assistance for pancreatitis management. The Pancreas: Biology, Pathobiology, and Illnesses is a comprehensive and authoritative resource that gives up-to-date information and guidance on the biology and diseases of the pancreas.

Pancreatitis and Its Complications.

Pancreatitis and Its Consequences is a medical textbook that focuses on the diagnosis, treatment, and management of pancreatitis and its complications. The textbook contains in-depth information on the causes, symptoms, and risk factors for pancreatitis, as well as the different complications that can result from the condition. The textbook is intended for healthcare professionals, including gastroenterologists, surgeons, and specialists in the field of pancreatology. The textbook contains thorough information on diagnostic tests, medicinal and surgical therapies, and postoperative care, making it a helpful resource for people seeking information and assistance for pancreatitis therapy. Pancreatitis and Its Consequences is a comprehensive and authoritative resource that gives up-to-date information and recommendations on the diagnosis, treatment, and management of pancreatitis and its complications.

CHAPTER 15

Conclusion: The Benefits of a Nourishing Diet for Managing Pancreatitis.

Pancreatitis is a disorder that affects the pancreas, an organ found in the upper region of the belly. The pancreas is important for manufacturing digestive enzymes and hormones that regulate blood sugar levels. When the pancreas becomes inflamed, digestion enzymes are activated within the organ, leading to damage to the tissue and adjacent organs. Pancreatitis can be acute, meaning that it comes on abruptly and aggressively, or it can be chronic, indicating that it happens over a long period of time.

Managing pancreatitis can be a struggle, as it involves not only medical therapy but also lifestyle modifications, including dietary adjustments. A healthy diet can play a significant part in controlling pancreatitis, as it can help to alleviate symptoms, prevent future damage to the pancreas, and enhance overall health and wellbeing.

There are various benefits to following a healthy diet for controlling pancreatitis. Firstly, a healthy diet can help minimize symptoms such as abdominal pain, nausea, and vomiting. By consuming a diet that is low in fat and high in fiber, patients can help to lessen the strain on the pancreas, which can help to reduce inflammation and improve recovery.

Furthermore, a healthy diet can help prevent further pancreatic injury By consuming a diet that is low in fat and high in fiber, patients can help minimize the quantity of digestive enzymes that are produced by the pancreas. This can help limit the danger of future damage to the organ and reduce the risk of developing chronic pancreatitis.

Moreover, a healthy diet can help to enhance general health and wellbeing. By consuming a diet that is rich in nutrients, patients can help maintain the health of various organs and systems in the body. For example, a diet that is high in antioxidants can help minimize the risk of acquiring various health disorders, such as heart disease and cancer.

There are numerous dietary recommendations for patients with pancreatitis. Patients should attempt to consume a diet that is low in fat and high in fiber. This can help minimize the stress on the pancreas and encourage recovery. They should attempt to consume a diet that is rich in nutrients, including vitamins, minerals, and antioxidants. This can help to support the health of various organs and systems in the body.

Finally, patients should attempt to consume a diet that is balanced and varied. This means that patients should attempt to consume a wide range of various foods, including fruits, vegetables, whole grains, lean proteins, and healthy fats. By consuming a balanced and diverse diet, patients may help to ensure that they are obtaining all of the nutrients that they need to maintain their health and wellness.

In conclusion, a healthy diet can play a key role in managing pancreatitis. By adopting a diet that is low in fat, high in fiber, and rich in nutrients, patients can help minimize symptoms, avoid additional damage to the pancreas, and promote overall health and wellbeing. By consuming a balanced and diverse diet, patients may help to ensure that they are obtaining all of the nutrients that they need to maintain their health and wellness. If you are suffering from pancreatitis, it is vital to consult with your healthcare professional to design a nutritional plan that is ideal for you.